D0615646

PEOPLE COUNT

PEOPLE COUNT

CONTACT-TRACING APPS AND PUBLIC HEALTH

SUSAN LANDAU

The MIT Press
Cambridge, Massachusetts
London, England

This book was set in Minion and Neue Haas Grotesk by Jen Jackowitz.
Printed and bound in the United States of America.

Library of Congress Cataloging-in-Publication Data

Names: Landau, Susan Eva, author.
Title: People count : contact-tracing apps and public health / Susan Landau.
Description: Cambridge, Massachusetts : The MIT Press, [2021] | Includes
    bibliographical references and index.
Identifiers: LCCN 2020054454 | ISBN 9780262045711 (hardcover)
Subjects: MESH: Contact Tracing | Mobile Applications | Pandemics—
    prevention & control | Privacy | Computer Security | Socioeconomic Factors
Classification: LCC RA418 | NLM WA 110 | DDC 362.1—dc23
LC record available at https://lccn.loc.gov/2020054454

10 9 8 7 6 5 4 3 2 1

To the memory of Joseph Rotblat, who taught me the responsibilities of being a scientist, and Chiune Sugihara, who saved my grandfather's life

CONTENTS

PREFACE

In mid-February some colleagues and I flew to Brussels to brief European Union policymakers on a report on encryption policy we had prepared as part of a Carnegie Endowment for International Peace project. In our forty-eight hours there, we briefed members of the European Commission and European Parliament and held an evening convening with stakeholders from the government, industry, civil society, and academia. We managed a stop at a famed chocolate shop and a dinner out that included Belgian beer. As I headed home, one of the airline personnel asked me if I had been exposed to the coronavirus. "No," I laughed, "I have only been in Brussels." Little did I, or almost anyone else, know that the disease was already widely circulating in Europe.[1]

I flew home, then two days later went with my husband to visit our son in Austin. It was a tiring trip—as travel often is. Our son and daughter-in-law love to walk. I do too, but I am twice their age. We walked extensively through parks and interesting Austin neighborhoods. That Sunday night, I fell into bed, exhausted. The next morning, my husband flew back home, while I continued on to a planned trip to California. Tuesday morning, my throat was a bit sore. By the end of the day, my symptoms had blossomed into a cold. That was unfortunate, as I was staying with two sets of friends and I had numerous appointments.

Aside from socializing with my friends, this trip put me in the midst of thousands of strangers. Two of my appointments had been set up by Tufts University, my employer, to advise me on a program we were setting up on cyber security and policy. I was also speaking on a panel on encryption policy at a huge computer security meeting of 36,000 people. Two days later, I spoke at a smaller meeting organized by UC Berkeley's law school on technology and the law. It was no time to be ill, but ill I was, with sneezes, coughs, a runny nose, an upset stomach, and fever.[2]

You know where this is going; I didn't, and neither did anyone else. I was surprised by the upset stomach—I'm always careful about what I eat when I travel—but not so surprised by fever; I can develop a fever at the drop of a hat. I was disconcerted by the fatigue that sent me to bed at 3:30 on Thursday afternoon and 6 pm on Friday. But even though I skipped the Berkeley banquet, I managed to give my two presentations. And because I was sneezing, I kept far away from people. No one on the panels, no one I had coffee with, and no one I visited fell ill—at least as far as I know.

I flew home. I was better the following week, though oddly and frighteningly, I coughed up blood a few times. But I was in Boston and my physician, a new one whom I had not yet met, was in western Massachusetts, where I live. I made an appointment for the following week in case the symptom persisted. This was now the first week in March, and coronavirus disease 2019 (COVID-19) was beginning to claim more of the American press's attention. More than once, I checked the website of the Centers for Disease Control and Prevention (CDC). But with the exception of the blood, all my symptoms pointed to a cold.

I had another busy week: Washington, DC, for an encryption policy briefing and running a two-day student symposium on cybersecurity policy at Tufts. Afterwards, my husband and I managed to squeeze in dinner with two old friends, biostatisticians at the Harvard Medical School and Brown University. They spoke very differently about the potential seriousness and danger of COVID-19 than did the news stories and CDC site. Two days later, I returned home as planned to western Massachusetts. It was March 10, and I was now recovered from my cold. I saw the doctor, who said my slightly painful ear—the only remaining symptom of the dreadful cold—would heal on its own.

Two weeks later, the *New York Times* published an article that caught my attention, titled "Lost Sense of Smell May Be Peculiar Clue to Coronavirus Infection." I'd had that symptom—anosmia—when I arrived in California. Two weeks after that, another *New York Times* story changed my understanding of my illness.[3]

"Google Searches Can Help Us Find Emerging COVID-19 Outbreaks," wrote Seth Stephens-Davidowitz in an opinion column. Stephens-Davidowitz said that searches for "my eyes hurt" had risen in exactly the parts of the United States that were experiencing high COVID-19 rates. One has to be careful about such data—earlier claims that searches for "flu" could be an early indicator of flu outbreaks, even ahead of CDC data, were incorrect—but this hint was later borne out by scientific studies that showed eye symptoms similar to conjunctivitis in a small percentage of COVID-19 patients. Bingo! I had spent the first several days in California looking at my eyes in the mirror, for they had been bothering me and I was concerned that I had conjunctivitis (I didn't).[4]

It was now over five weeks since I had fallen ill; it was impossible to get tested for COVID-19. Indeed, even when I was sick, it would have been impossible for me to get tested: I didn't fit the criterion of having been to China or of having been in contact with someone who had. And while that is one of the multiple reasons the number of US cases exploded, it's also one of the factors that led to this book.

A second motivation to write this book relates to my research in cybersecurity. For twenty-five years, I've worked on issues of encryption and wiretap policy. This work has brought me to Brussels; Washington, DC; and other places, but it's also led me to ask important questions about the use of communications metadata. At just the moment in the spring of 2020 that the coronavirus was rapidly spreading around the world, I was exploring the types of private information one could discern from communications metadata. Meanwhile, I was hearing smart people propose using GPS data to track individuals with the disease—even though the coronavirus spreads best indoors, where GPS doesn't work well. I wrote a blog post to clarify this issue. As I learned that COVID-19 can spread from people who have no symptoms, I wrote another post on the efficacy of contact-tracing apps. Then, along with Christy Lopez and Laura Moy, I wrote a third on equity issues raised by using mobile apps for contact tracing. At that point, MIT Press sought a book on contact-tracing apps. Here I was.[5]

There was a third reason for this book, too: what was occurring in my hometown. I've lived in the countryside of New England for half my life, but I was born in New York City. That wonderful, dynamic, ethnically diverse city made me who I am. I am a first-generation American, the daughter of two people who never went to college (my father never finished high school). Yet I have a PhD from one of the best educational institutions in the world. Smarts got me there, but the education and encouragement I received from New York City public schools allowed me to flourish. For that I am forever grateful.

New York City gave me many things—a lifelong love of theater and the New York City Ballet, a wonderful math and science education in high school, enrichment in Saturday science courses for high school students at Columbia University, the 92nd Street Y where I heard Marianne Moore speak, sculpture classes at MOMA, and so much more. The city also gave me a tremendous appreciation for the diversity of its people. I may love living in the country, but I never feel so alive as when I walk down New York streets and ride its subways.

In the spring of 2020, that world was being torn apart. COVID-19 was hitting people of color and poor neighborhoods far worse than it was the wealthy reaches of Manhattan. It was killing people, and it was potentially killing my city. I'm not an epidemiologist or a medical doctor, and I couldn't help cure the people who were ill. But if I, working in security and surveillance, could shed light on what kinds of protection contact-tracing apps can and can't provide, I will have given back a tiny bit to the city that has given me so much. Hence this book.

I am completing this book in early fall 2020; even as I write, the ground underneath contact-tracing apps is shifting. The details of the apps will undoubtedly be different by the time this book appears, and different again six months after its publication. If I focused precisely on what TraceTogether, Aarogya Setu, or any other app does or doesn't do, I will have written a book that is dated by the time the manuscript leaves my hands. Instead, I have sought to write a book that captures the essence of current contact-tracing and exposure-notification apps, discusses their limitations, and addresses the important social and political issues their use raises. Those issues will not disappear with version 2.0 or 3.1, even though the details of any given app may differ slightly. If the discussion I present provides some insight for the policy choices we must make as we fight this pandemic or the next one—and the next one will come—then I will have succeeded in my mission.

1 INTRODUCTION

We are surrounded by germs. They fill the oceans and the soil, cover the outside of our skin, and inhabit our bodies. They are tiny—microscopic—and they come in a wondrous variety of forms: prions, viruses, bacteria, protozoa, and fungi.

Prions, the most recently discovered type of germs, are twisted forms of proteins that cause such illnesses as mad cow disease. Viruses are not alive; they can't even replicate unless they get inside a host cell and use the cell's replication machinery to reproduce. Bacteria are single-celled organisms that lack a nucleus but contain DNA. Protozoans are also single-celled, but unlike bacteria, they have a nucleus and other internal membranes. Fungi are organisms such as mushrooms that reproduce by spores; they can cause such mundane problems as athlete's foot.

We humans are vastly outnumbered by the microscopic world, at a scale that's difficult to comprehend. As a science writer for *Nature* put it, there are 100 million times more bacteria in the ocean alone than the number of stars known in 2011.[1]

Many of these microscopic organisms are necessary for life. Indeed, plants use bacteria to convert atmospheric nitrogen into a usable form, and we humans depend on the bacteria in our digestive systems to break down and absorb the proteins, fats, and carbohydrates we eat. The viruses that replicate within and attack bacteria—bacteriophages—prevent certain types of harmful bacteria from entering our bodies through the soft tissues of our nose and mouth. Fungi produce delicious foods we know and love, including beer, bread, blue cheese, and truffles. More importantly, they also produce penicillin. And protozoa, which include amoeba and paramecia, eat bacteria and help the soil decompose; without them, we couldn't produce food.

But some germs kill us. Some target the lungs, kidney, or brain; others launch multipronged attacks against multiple parts of an organism. Their mode of transmission varies, too. Some germs travel through the air or through the exchange of body fluids, while others can be picked up from a surface on which they've landed or from contaminated water or food. Germs can be transmitted from person to person, or they may require an intermediate host. Malaria, for instance, travels between people via the bite of a mosquito. Germs are a complex adversary.

From the bubonic plague to influenza to AIDS, human societies have struggled to understand, fight, and end pandemics caused by germs. The challenges posed by COVID-19 may appear unprecedented, but most pandemics have a few things in common. And humans have learned how to use that in tackling the diseases.

People took on this fight against deadly germs well before they understood anything about viruses, bacteria, or protozoa. In the eleventh century, the Persian physician Ibn Sana observed that tuberculosis spread directly from person to person, even as the source of transmission remained a mystery. In 1668, an Italian physician, Francisco Redi, put fresh meat into three jars—a sealed one, an open one, and one covered with cloth netting—and showed that maggots appeared only in the open-air jar. His experiment showed that maggots had to come from somewhere—that is, they could not spontaneously generate—but it didn't resolve the mystery of what caused disease.[2]

Less than a decade later, a Dutch shopkeeper studying rainwater and dental plaque provided another clue. While Galileo Galilei was busy training telescopes on the heavens, Antonie van Leeuwenhoek ground lenses to look at the microscopic world. He found dancing "small animals"—bacteria—within the seemingly clear rainwater and plaque. The teeming world of microscopic creatures living in, on, and around us appeared extraordinary—and indeed it was. Leeuwenhoek's microscope showed that we were supporting entire communities of living creatures on and in our bodies. But Leeuwenhoek was a naturalist, not a physician; his studies could reveal microbes' existence, but not their effects.

As the centuries passed, doctors and scientists continued to search for the causes of disease. In 1854, British physician John Snow combined knowledge of both people and place to stop a cholera outbreak in a crowded London neighborhood. The most popular theory at the time was that diseases spread through "miasma"—bad air. Snow didn't buy it, in part because of an observation he had made five years earlier: residents of adjoining houses, who presumably breathed the same air, could experience very different rates of cholera infection.[3]

What Snow had observed was that cholera would appear only after someone came from somewhere where the disease was present. Snow posited that the disease came from swallowing some kind of material that then multiplied inside the body; he became convinced that the disease was transmitted by water. He began studying water samples in the neighborhood of the outbreak.[4]

The outbreak had begun the night of August 31. Snow quickly realized that deaths were concentrated in the area surrounding the Broad Street water pump. He collected drinking water samples on September 3, but these contained relatively little organic matter. Later samples had much more. When he reported this to the neighborhood Board of Guardians—essentially the district's government—they immediately shut down the pump. Snow did not discover the bacterium responsible for the epidemic, but the connection he drew between the pump and the deaths stopped the cholera outbreak and changed the practice of public health.[5]

But what had caused the cholera? Snow didn't figure that out, but an Italian researcher did. In 1854, a year before Snow's investigation into the Broad Street pump, Filippo Pacini had found the comma-shaped bacteria that caused cholera (though he didn't show that it did so). But Pacini's paper lay ignored for decades, not the first or last time that correct scientific answers are overlooked. The bacteria's more famous discoverer was Robert Koch, the founder of bacteriology.

Koch, a German physician, was obsessed with finding the causes of diseases. He started with anthrax, a disease that could kill a healthy flock of animals in a matter of days—and then kill the farmer, too. Looking at the blood of dead sheep and cows, Koch noticed that the blood of infected animals contained microscopic rods. When he infected live mice with blood that contained these rods, the mice got infected too.[6]

Koch had discovered the anthrax bacillus. In time, he would also identify the bacterium that caused tuberculosis, and the one for cholera. But far more important than those discoveries were Koch's contributions to the germ theory of disease. Koch postulated that the link between bacterial organisms and diseases was both specific and necessary. The anthrax bacillus could no more cause TB than could bad air, but unless the anthrax bacillus was present, there was no anthrax. Koch's work remains fundamental for how we treat infectious diseases.

Ending a plague requires more than medication: we need to stop spread. And for that, as John Snow demonstrated, we need data. Although the type of evidence differs, history offers ample data on the nature of pandemics: how they start, how they spread, how they end. Each disease begins as a mystery: what it is and how it spreads.

The history of the flu, which may be the world's oldest pandemic, is instructive. Some historians believe that flu epidemics occurred in India as early as four millennia ago. Long before airplanes and globalization enabled the global spread of disease, flu pandemics affected Asia, Europe, Africa, and the Americas. Relatively accurate records since an outbreak in Asia in 1580 indicate that flu has caused at least forty-six pandemics or serious epidemics in the past five centuries.[7]

Flu is an upper respiratory disease, which means that we spread it to each other by coughing and sneezing. Once you've had a particular strain of flu, you develop immunity to it—but there's a catch. The flu is caused by a virus, and like all viruses, its genes mutate. Most mutations are minor, enabling anyone who has developed immunity to a strain to retain it against a close version of the disease. But over the space of a year, a flu changes enough that a person doesn't necessarily have immunity to the most common strain in circulation.[8]

Flu is zoonotic; that is, it can infect multiple animals as well as people. This is one of the reasons the disease has proved so dangerous for humans. The virus can mutate within different species—birds, pigs, horses—then come back to infect us. This ability to jump back and forth between humans and other animals increases the virus's capacity for mutation. When new versions make the jump from animal to human, they spread quickly around the world. Indeed, avian and swine flus have repeatedly done so.[9]

Flu normally kills 0.1 percent of those infected, but mortality rates vary dramatically according to the strain. The Spanish flu, a particularly deadly variety, killed approximately 10 percent of those infected when it raged across the globe between 1918 and 1920. Both death rates are extremely low compared to those of the Black Death, the fourteenth-century outbreak of bubonic plague that killed between a third and a half of the population of Europe.

Bubonic plague is caused by *Yersinia pestis*, a bacterium transmitted by fleas. The bacteria are present around the world; rodents, especially rats, carry the fleas that transmit the disease.

Although the *Yersinia pestis* bacterium still circulates in rodents and fleas, bubonic plague no longer represents a serious threat to humans. For one thing, the infection can be cured through quick antibiotic treatment (rapid response is critical; 60 percent of untreated sufferers die). And unless someone develops pneumonic plague—plague in the lungs—people don't transmit the disease to one other. Eliminating the vector of disease—the fleas or the rats—ends its spread.[10]

Similar tales of surprise and fear could be told about any number of epidemics, but let's focus instead on their most salient common features. Lethal diseases emerge from time to time; they can produce dramatic social effects in addition to grief and suffering. Over time, one of two things happens. Either the disease becomes endemic and we learn to live with it, or we figure out how to stop its spread.

Different factors affect whether a disease leads to an outbreak, an epidemic, or worse. One crucial aspect of spread is a disease's contagiousness. Epidemiologists use R_0, pronounced "R naught," to represent the "reproduction number" of a disease. An R_0 less than one means that, on average, each infection will result in less than one additional infection. The disease, in other words, will die out. If R_0 equals one, then each infection causes, on average, an additional one. The disease will not die out, but neither will it cause an epidemic. If R_0 is greater than one, however, each infection causes, on average, more than one infection. These are ripe conditions for an outbreak, an epidemic, or possibly even a pandemic.

Even for a given disease, R_0 varies with environment and human behavior. Respiratory illnesses are affected by weather; smallpox and flu, for example, spread less during damp periods. An infectious disease spreads more easily in the crowded immigrant dormitories of Singapore than on the sparsely populated pampas of Patagonia. For HIV/AIDS, R_0 varies with people's sexual behavior and drug use. And when there's "herd immunity," when most of the population has immunity to the disease, R_0 is lower.

R_0 estimates for COVID-19 were all over the map, from a low of 2.2 to a high of 5.7. The size of this range shouldn't be surprising. There's much we don't yet understand about COVID-19. Epidemiologists determine R_0 based on accurate data. At the beginning of the pandemic, cases were often misdiagnosed—and often not tested—due to stringent testing criteria and an incomplete list of symptoms. The fact that the disease can be spread by people who are asymptomatic only complicated epidemiologists' ability to pin down COVID-19's R_0. With better data, epidemiologists now believe R_0 to be between 2 and 3 in the absence of any types of controls such as masks and social distancing.[11]

High R_0s are a reason for concern, but they do not convey the full story of an epidemic's impact. The R_0 for measles is astounding, ranging from somewhere between 12 and 18 depending on community immunity. Smallpox has a much lower R_0—somewhere between 3.5 and 6—but is more dangerous than measles because its death rate is 30 percent compared to measles's 0.2 percent. The legendary Spanish flu of 1918 had a relatively mild—at least in comparison to the numbers we've mentioned so far—R_0 of 1.7–2. Yet the Spanish flu, with its 10 percent mortality rate, killed at least 50 million people, or around 3 percent of the entire world population.[12]

The way that a disease spreads matters nearly as much as its level of contagion. To cause a pandemic, a disease must spread efficiently as well as directly between people. A disease that kills its host too quickly—before the host has managed to infect others—will itself die out. And the disease can't kill everyone; it needs hosts to survive to attack another day.

Measles checks all the boxes for a potential pandemic. Its high R_0 is explained by the ease of which it is transmitted, either through airborne droplets containing the virus or through rash secretions. Up to 90 percent of people exposed to measles develop the disease. The disease can produce serious complications, including death. That's why the measles vaccine has been so important in eliminating this childhood disease in much of the world.

The habits of modern human life greatly increase the risk of global pandemics. By concentrating people, urbanization provides easy paths for diseases to spread from human to human. Poor sanitation and crowded conditions create spaces for disease to thrive. A classic example is tuberculosis, a curable disease that flourished in the early twentieth-century slums of New York City and continues to do so in those of India, China, Indonesia, the

Philippines, Pakistan, Nigeria, Bangladesh, and South Africa. And with air routes crisscrossing the planet, we have reduced the time in which a disease can spread from years to hours.[13]

The recent spread of cities into previously wild areas raises the risk of new infections. Zoonotic diseases are not new, but large concentrations of people now live in close proximity to wild animals. These creatures provide a rich pool of new pathogens.

Through trade, travel, and geographic expansion, humans have turned epidemics into pandemics. Germs need carriers. Bubonic plague traveled along the Silk Route from Asia to Europe in animal hosts, while West Nile virus made its way from Africa to Europe through migrating birds. In early 2020, foreign travelers fleeing Wuhan spread severe acute respiratory syndrome 2 (SARS-CoV-2), the coronavirus that causes COVID-19, across the globe.

From its first appearance in December 2019, COVID-19 has stretched our ability to cope with infectious disease. It is thought to have emerged from an animal host, in a crowded city and transportation hub, with confusing or even no symptoms, and is highly infectious. The leading US expert on infectious disease, Dr. Anthony Fauci, ticked off the timeline: "First notice at the end of December [2019], hit China in January, hit the rest of the world in February, March, April, May, early June." COVID spread like wildfire. Even for someone who spent his career imagining the dangers of a new pandemic, this disease turned out to be Fauci's "worst nightmare."[14]

Sometimes, in the battle of humans versus germs, the humans win. The elimination of smallpox, a disease that had caused epidemics for millennia, represents a victory of medicine and international cooperation. We don't know when humankind first suffered smallpox; there is "tantalizing speculation" that it was as early as the tenth century BCE. The symptoms of smallpox include characteristic red spots that become small blisters that first fill with clear fluid, later changing over to pus. The lucky two out of three who survive are left with scars on their faces, arms, and legs.[15]

Highly contagious and thriving in densely populated areas, smallpox was endemic in European cities by the fifteenth century. Those who survived were immune, a fact that changed the course of history. When sixteenth-century European explorers brought smallpox and measles to the New World, Native Americans had never been exposed to either disease. The epidemics that followed ravaged the native population.[16]

Thanks to several centuries of vaccination and an ambitious eradication program, smallpox no longer poses a threat in ordinary life. Vaccination against smallpox was practiced in the Ottoman Empire in the sixteenth century, using a technique that appears to have been first developed in China or India. This method, variolation, which involves inoculating someone with live virus from smallpox patients, had a death rate of 1–2 percent. In the late eighteenth century, the English physician Edward Jenner developed a vaccine based on cowpox, a milder form of the illness that infected milkmaids and left them immune to smallpox. His vaccine inoculated against the disease without variolation's relatively high death rate.[17]

The possibility of vaccination reduced the number of smallpox fatalities, but the disease did not disappear. Instead, by the end of the nineteenth century, the disease was everywhere, endemic in most nations of the world. Half a century later, public health authorities floated an audacious plan to eradicate it.[18]

That this even seemed possible was the result of the disease's disappearance in the 1940s and 1950s from Europe and the Americas. In Europe, Canada, Mexico, and South America this occurred through mass vaccination, while in the UK and US, it was done through controlling known outbreaks and selective vaccination. In 1959 the World Health Organization (WHO) launched a global eradication program that would attempt to vaccinate at least 80 percent of people in places with endemic smallpox. The program failed for a variety of reasons, ranging from a lack of funding to Cold War tensions to the politics of decolonization. But when WHO took up a second approach in 1967, it succeeded.[19]

Studies in Pakistan and elsewhere showed that the spread of smallpox could be stopped by focusing on case surveillance and containment (yes, "surveil" is the word health professionals use). With smallpox, it is easy to tell when someone is sick: infected people develop pocks on their face or other extremities. Instead of vaccinating everyone, the idea was to eliminate the spread of disease from one person to another. Such a technique can work with diseases that are spread through interpersonal contact and have no animal reservoirs.[20]

This public health approach, typically referred to as "surveil and contain," requires accurate reporting of the appearance of the disease. Before WHO could do anything else, it had to assure that reporting was accurate. Prior to the campaign, clinics and hospitals only documented the cases that came to them, which meant that they were missing ninety-nine cases out of a hundred. The patients hadn't been turning up because the health centers couldn't help them.[21]

Surveil and contain relies on contact tracing, that is, identifying people who have been in contact with an infected person. But in the smallpox campaign, public health authorities took surveil and contain a step further, to something called "ring vaccination." Everyone in close contact with a smallpox patient was to be vaccinated, as was everyone in close contact with the contacts. The strategy worked, with the last case of endemic smallpox occurring in October 1977.[22]

Eradicating an infectious disease is the exception, not the rule. The disease can't have animal reservoirs that would allow it to reappear in mutated form. There must be obvious ways to discern when someone is infected, and cases must be accurately reported. There must be a vaccine. And there must be either a high rate of vaccination in the population or, as was the case with the end of smallpox, a sufficiently low spread that ring vaccination can work.

The success story of smallpox contrasts sharply with the world's failure to end tuberculosis (TB). In this case, the stars did not align, despite the fact that the disease can be cured by antibiotics. TB, a disease that has been with us since at least the time of the pharaohs, is widespread; a quarter of the world's population is infected, although only 5–10 percent of infected people will go on to develop the disease. Once a disease is present in so many people, the usual methods of public health—test, trace, isolate—become harder to implement. And over time, treatment has become less easy than it was; the disease has developed strains that are resistant to multiple antibiotics. Today, TB kills more people annually than any other infectious disease; people with weakened immune systems, including those with HIV/AIDS, are especially vulnerable.[23]

Diseases like TB and COVID-19 in which asymptomatic people can spread infection are particularly challenging to control. Another of these diseases is typhoid, a bacterial infection spread by eating or drinking food contaminated by fecal traces from the carrier. In the early twentieth century, public health authorities imprisoned an asymptomatic typhoid carrier and cook named Mary Mallon. Based on contact tracing and stool samples, public health authorities in New York accused

Mallon, an Irish immigrant, of infecting at least fifty-two people and killing at least two. Since there was no way to cure her infection, and since Mallon kept returning to work as a cook, public health authorities had her arrested and quarantined on North Brother Island twice—the second time for life. When there is no treatment for a disease, surveil and contain presents social and ethical dilemmas that public health authorities have yet to resolve.[24]

Aside from the question of vaccines, general prevalence, and the availability of treatment, public health authorities face a different problem when attempting to control sexually transmitted diseases like syphilis, gonorrhea, and HIV/AIDS (which is also transmitted through the blood). Surveil and contain only works when those infected are willing to share how they might have been infected and whom they might have passed the disease along to. Stigma, discrimination, gender expectations, the risk of arrest, and just plain personal privacy issues limit people's willingness to disclose information about their sexual partners, and this in turn limits authorities' ability to stop the spread of sexually transmitted diseases.

Pandemics end in various ways. The London cholera outbreak ended because John Snow traced the problem to water from the Broad Street pump—and got it shut down. Smallpox was eradicated by combining surveil and contain with ring vaccination. A pandemic can end because we find a cure, because we provide treatment even if we can't cure the underlying disease, or because we can vaccinate against it. But sometimes we are unable to contain the disease through any of these techniques. And then, unless you quarantine everyone—which is what Wuhan did in early 2020—you must find some way of locating those who have been exposed to the disease. That's contact tracing.

Contact tracing involves feet on the ground. Contact tracers interview people to find out the intimate details of their lives, including whom they spent time with or, in some cases, whom they had sex with. Contact tracers seek to learn where people spend their days. A tracer might have to tell someone to upend their lives, and their incomes, for a period of quarantine. The job is part detective, part social worker, and part medical investigator. It's labor-intensive and highly privacy-invasive. And it's never been tried before in a situation of wide community spread of a highly contagious respiratory disease.

Contact tracing also necessarily infringes upon the privacy and autonomy of individuals, albeit in order to end an epidemic. The questions a contact tracer asks constitute an invasion of privacy—and not for the purpose of protecting the individual, but to protect the public's health. Under the circumstances, it's not surprising that contact tracers have sometimes struggled to convince the public to participate. Yet we also know that, when it works right, contact tracing is one of the most effective tools of public health there is.[25]

2 STOPPING A PANDEMIC

By the time a smallpox outbreak occurred in Bradford, England, in January 1962, the country was largely free of the disease. The authorities first noticed something strange in Bradford when a cook from Bradford's Children's Hospital was admitted to a "fever hospital" (a hospital used for isolating those with severe diseases). The cook's blood sample indicated a severe viral infection, with unusual damage to the blood cells. But what kind of virus?[1]

The hematologist, Derrick Tovey, soon received a second blood sample from a person at a different Bradford hospital who was experiencing the same unusual and life-threatening problems. This patient was so ill that he died even as doctors were examining his blood sample.[2]

Tovey turned to textbooks to resolve the mystery. A 1925 manual suggested smallpox. With a lab confirmation slated to take two days, the doctors needed to immediately find out how the cook had been infected. Then they had to trace that patient's contacts.[3]

The original case—what epidemiologists call the "index case"—turned out to be a nine-year-old girl who had been on the wards at the Children's Hospital. She had emigrated from Pakistan with her parents in mid-December and had fallen ill soon after her arrival. She had been vaccinated against small-pox in Karachi, but apparently the vaccine didn't take. When the child died, the autopsy attributed her death to a combination of malaria and septicemia. But the child also had smallpox.[4]

The girl had died on December 23, but the Bradford doctors did not realize that smallpox was circulating in the area until January 11. The delay in diagnosis meant that all four hospitals in the city and one outside were "infected" by smallpox as patients had been transferred between them. There were not only "first-generation" infections resulting from exposure to the original case—including children on the hospital ward, the cook, and the pathologist who conducted the postmortem—but also second-generation infections from the first-generation cases. A potential 1,400 people had been exposed, and all needed to be contacted. Even with the scope of this exposure, the British medical establishment did not suggest mass vaccination for a disease that had, after all, been largely absent from the British Isles since the 1930s. The British public, which had been resisting smallpox vaccination of infants, now saw risk differently and demanded access to vaccines. Within five days, five-sixths of Bradford's population—250,000 people—were vaccinated.[5]

Just two months later, another possible smallpox outbreak erupted in a place where the disease had supposedly been eradicated. This time, the case appeared in Farmington, New Mexico. No one involved had traveled from abroad, so confirmation of smallpox would mean that a disease thought to have been eliminated from North America was, in fact, still present.[6]

No one examining the ten-month-old baby in Farmington—neither the resident physician nor the CDC's Epidemic Intelligence Service (EIS) doctor who flew in for a consult—had ever seen smallpox. Like Tovey, they had to consult an older text-book. The baby's lesions were atypical for the disease, but the hospital's initial lab tests could not rule out smallpox. As the doctors awaited definitive lab results from CDC, state and local health departments began contact tracing. Identifying the baby's contacts for the previous three weeks, and those people's contacts, would be necessary to contain an outbreak. In contrast to Bradford, public health authorities recommended and began preparing for a vaccination program.[7]

By day three, the baby had new spots. Now the situation became clear: the child had herpes, not smallpox. The baby was suffering from multiple diseases—pneumonia, severe thrush enteritis, herpes—and was recovering from measles, a routine childhood illness in the era before widespread measles vaccination. There was no smallpox and no public health emergency. The measles spots had lain on top of herpes sores, confusing diagnosis.[8]

Two issues stand out from these stories. The first is the complexity of diagnosis. In Bradford, doctors missed the index child's smallpox. In Farmington, herpes added confusion to what should have been an easy determination of a child's illness.

Diagnosis can be difficult when a disease is unusual or unexpected. The difficulty increases when a patient has multiple infections whose overlapping symptoms hide an essential aspect of a particular illness. And diagnosis can be particularly challenging if a disease is new and its symptoms are not fully known.

The complexity of diagnosis has become part of the story of COVID-19. The first patients diagnosed with the disease presented with pneumonia of unknown cause. By mid-January 2020, fever, dry cough, and fatigue were also known to be symptoms. In mid-March, people who were worried that they had been exposed were being asked if they had lost their sense of smell and taste. More symptoms have accumulated since then.

In late January, we also learned that someone infected with COVID-19 can be infectious before developing symptoms, that is, while pre-symptomatic. Still later we discovered the disease could be spread by asymptomatic carriers.[9]

Both of these stories also illustrate the importance of contact tracing in containing an outbreak. If a community has resistance to a disease, either through previous exposure or vaccination, then the rate of infection, R_0, is low. This is the case, for example, in communities where the disease is endemic. But in the absence of herd immunity, a disease with a high R_0 needs to be contained in other ways—and that's contact tracing.

Contact tracing is a multistep process that requires not just tracing contacts, but also getting them tested, isolated, and treated—if treatment is possible. The ultimate goal is stopping the spread of the disease. Each epidemic-causing disease differs in how it spreads, when it spreads, and what sort of isolation and quarantine is needed to stop its spread. Epidemiologists solve the mystery of a disease's trajectory, while contact tracers put that knowledge to use in stopping it.

There's something else I should mention about Bradford's smallpox epidemic. The Bradford outbreak occurred against the backdrop of increasing British resentment against immigrants from its former colonies. A small manufacturing city in Yorkshire, Bradford's population of 300,000 included an immigrant population of 10,000, largely from Pakistan, India, and the West Indies. Days before the outbreak, the *Daily Mail*, one of England's right-wing tabloids, editorialized, "KEEP OUT THE GERMS," claiming, "They came to Britain by air, walked in without any trouble, *and were at once a peril to the population*." When smallpox was confirmed, some national papers ran xenophobic headlines, like "City in Fear!" and "Keep Out the Pakistanis." This sort of response to the appearance of a new or unexpected disease is, unfortunately, not uncommon.[10]

Every pandemic is perceived as coming from somewhere else. Syphilis is perhaps the most famous example. The Turks called syphilis the disease of the Franks (Christians); the Germans called it the French disease; the French called it the Neapolitan disease; the Italians referred to it as the French or Spanish disease. The Spanish said it came from Española (the island that is now the Dominican Republic and Haiti). In northern India, Hindus and Muslims blamed each other for the disease. Some have tried to pin the disease's arrival in Europe on the New World, but there's also some evidence that syphilis—or a precursor of it—was present in Europe before the era of colonialization. No matter where it came from, we know for a fact that syphilis became significantly more virulent around the end of the fifteenth century.

The first indication of a syphilis infection is a small sore in the area where the bacteria entered the body. This sore usually appears on the genitals or anus, but it can also appear around the mouth, as syphilis is occasionally spread through kissing. This first evidence of infection typically appears about three weeks after exposure. Shortly thereafter, any visible indication of an infection disappears. A few weeks later, however, people infected with the disease begin to develop secondary syphilis. They may develop a non-itchy rash or pustules, or they may simply have muscle aches or a sore throat, or they may not have any visible symptoms at all. Either way, they can still infect others. If a woman infected with secondary syphilis is pregnant, she has a 40 percent chance of a miscarriage, stillbirth, or the baby dying shortly after birth. But the disease is not done yet: a sixth to a third of those with syphilis suffer a final, more wretched stage. The disease attacks the brain, the eyes, and the nervous system.[11]

For centuries, mercury was the drug of choice for treating syphilis, but as a treatment it was less than ideal. Mercury is toxic; its use can cause patients to lose feeling in their extremities, lose their teeth, suffer kidney failure—or even death. When Salvarsan, an arsenic-based drug against syphilis, became available in the early 1910s, it was viewed as a great improvement. But the ghostlike nature of syphilis—invisible yet contagious—makes controlling it particularly difficult. Salvarsan took years to cure a patient, and many quit taking it when their symptoms disappeared. Feeling better but still contagious, these syphilis carriers went on to infect others.[12]

The result was a high level of syphilis infection. In the United States, 1 percent of military draftees for World War I had the disease. Putting young men on military bases or at war increased those numbers; between 1917 and 1919, nearly 400,000 soldiers were diagnosed with syphilis, gonorrhea, or chancroid (a bacterial infection affecting the genitals). By the 1930s, 5 percent of the entire US population was being treated for syphilis. The government preached sexual abstinence—especially to soldiers—but that approach didn't get very far. Sexually transmitted diseases (STDs) tend to thrive in wartime.[13]

Ridding the United States of the disease took a deep commitment from the highest ranks of the public health services, the 1943 discovery that penicillin could cure the disease, and a plan. Thomas Parran, named Surgeon General in 1934, developed a plan to find the cases, trace their contacts, and test and treat them. This was an excellent plan, except that it was paired with an appalling forty-year study that produced decades of distrust of public health authorities by the Black community. In Macon County, Alabama, the disease would be researched, rather than treated.[14]

In 1932, the US Public Health Service (USPHS) began a syphilis study, advertising that it would treat people with "bad blood." This was the "Tuskegee Study of Untreated Syphilis in the Black Male," a forty-year experiment on the effects of not treating syphilis. The subjects were 400 rural Black men, largely illiterate and desperately poor; they were chosen because they all had tertiary-stage syphilis that had never been treated.

The study was proposed by a PHS officer, Dr. Taliaferro Clark. A study conducted in Oslo before arsenic-based treatment had become available showed that latent syphilis was likely to cause cardiovascular damage, but not neurologic complications. So, Clark proposed this study, whose purpose was to discover if untreated syphilis produced the same effects in Black people as in whites.[15]

The men were promised free health care. Instead, they were provided with hot meals, a pretense of treatment, and burial payments. The men were never informed that they had syphilis, how the disease would progress, or, after 1943, that there was a cure. They believed their problems were due to "bad blood."

Hard as it may be to believe, this study was not hidden. Reports of the study's results were published now and then in scientific journals. Local physicians knew not to treat the study patients. When World War II broke out and draft boards ordered the A-1 registrants in the study to get treatment, study doctors arranged for the men to be deemed "not draft eligible" and thus eliminated from obtaining treatment. Yet no one—not the CDC, not the Public Health Service, not local doctors—publicly questioned the ethics of the study. Only after an Associated Press reporter uncovered the story in 1972 was the experiment halted. Somewhere between 28 and 100 men in the study died of syphilis; some number of wives were infected as well.[16]

The legacy of Parran's grand plan to eliminate syphilis is mixed. On the one hand, by combining contact tracing and treatment, the USPHS dropped the syphilis numbers for white and Black populations. On the other, the agency sponsored a gruesome public health experiment on a group of 400 poverty-stricken Black men, depriving them of proper health care and treatment in the name of science.[17]

The negative impact of the Tuskegee study on Black people's health extended beyond the men and their families. It sowed mistrust in doctors and public health among the older local Black population living nearby (as well as those who had moved away). Middle-aged and older Black men went to the doctor less often—and that led to a likely shortened life expectancy of one and a half years. More broadly, it sharply amplified a distrust born from decades of racism. People of color in the United States have long faced disparities in health care, both in access to services and in treatment. The result of poorer medical care is shorter, less healthy lives, perpetuating disparities between these groups and other Americans. Tuskegee made this situation worse in a different way.[18]

The contact-tracing portion of Parran's plan came into being after the explosion of syphilis cases following World War II. In 1948 the federal government began training Public Health Advisers (PHAs). These workers were asked to combine several skills that neither doctors nor nurses necessarily possessed. They needed an understanding of the science of sexually transmitted diseases, an ability to recognize it, and the persistence to track down infected syphilis patients (many of whom did not want to be found). They also had to have that right mix of empathy and insistence to extract the names of sexual contacts from even the most reluctant of infected patients. And because it was hard to get some patients to come in for testing, they also had to know how to draw blood.[19]

The PHAs could take blood samples, but they weren't providing treatment. They were contact tracers, whose job it was to educate the patients about syphilis, then tactfully draw out the information about contacts. Their role was to inform a syphilis patient or contact about the disease, how it was transmitted, what the symptoms were, and what the options for treatment were.[20]

Interviewing a syphilis patient was a process. Since contact tracers first had to put the patient at ease, they took their time. They began by finding out who the person was, trying to plumb their character to figure out how and what to ask. Then the contact tracer would make sure that they had the right phone number and the right address so that they could follow up, if necessary. Only then would the contact tracer work around to getting detailed information about the patient's sexual contacts. The contact tracer was part social worker, part medical investigator, always seeking to establish trust. If a contact tracer was meeting with one of the contacts rather than a person with a known infection, they would inform the person that they might have been infected with syphilis and would offer to arrange testing.[21]

PHAs practiced role playing before they went out into the field. Dick Conlon, a CDC syphilis contact tracer who worked in Ohio, Michigan, and Minnesota, said he learned "to elicit accurate information from even the most belligerent patients." Contact tracers were trained to be patient but insistent. Like any good investigator, a contact tracer would return to the question of who their sexual contacts were if a patient didn't answer the first time, and then return to the question again. Often another try would do the trick. Contact tracers learned to ask open-ended questions and to actively listen so as to engage the patient and draw out more information.[22]

The syphilis PHAs were very skilled at drawing out information. David Sencer, a physician who later became director of the CDC, recalled a time when he examined a patient with secondary syphilis. During a half-hour exam and conversation, the patient revealed a single contact to Sencer: her husband. When the PHA tried again, the patient revealed thirteen contacts in a half-hour conversation.[23]

Even so, and perhaps inevitably, a contact's answers were sometimes wrong or misleading on details large and small. Contact tracers would walk the streets looking at mailboxes until they found the right person. And sometimes the work was dangerous. Conlon recalled his attempts to track down some prostitutes who worked a rough neighborhood in Detroit: "I'd go in early afternoon to the Anderson's Gardens [a bar], and I'd copy down the pay phone numbers. At 11, 12 at night, I would call and ask for Margo or Rita—and I would arrange to meet them [the next day] at the VD clinic." That was less dangerous for Conlon, Margo, and Rita.[24]

With the exception of the Tuskegee study, testing and treatment were part of the PHS's campaign. PHAs arranged rapid care for contacts, usually offering a same-day or next-day appointment in the clinic. If a patient opted for private care, the contact tracer would speak directly to the doctor about the recommended test and treatment—and then follow up afterwards to ensure that the patient had come in. Both testing and treatment were free at the public clinics; if a contact opted for private care, the government offered to provide the doctor with medications.

The contact tracers often went more than the extra mile. Conlon recalled a pregnant patient in Fremont, Ohio, who wanted to be treated by her obstetrician. But when Conlon called to confirm her treatment, the patient reported that the doctor "refused to treat her and sent her home without." Conlon got in his car in Toledo, where he and the clinic were based, and drove the thirty-five miles to Fremont to pick up the patient. He got her treated in Toledo, drove her home, and then interviewed her and arranged testing and treatment for her contacts as well. One hundred forty miles of driving to get a patient treated was part of a day's work for a contact tracer.[25]

In the 1940s, 1 percent of deaths in the United States were due to syphilis. The work of the PHAs brought those rates substantially down. And while it was penicillin that cured syphilis, what stopped syphilis's spread was finding the people who were ill and getting them help.[26]

The PHA efforts extended well beyond controlling the spread of syphilis. In 1957, the USPHS's VD Division was absorbed into the CDC. The PHAs' ability to "make things happen" also put them in the middle of the US polio immunization program; later, they would be brought into the international effort to eradicate smallpox. But that takes us far from our story. For contact tracers, the next big challenge was HIV/AIDS.

Contact tracing can't work without testing, but testing requires an understanding of what the disease is. The human immunodeficiency virus (HIV) started out as a mystery—and a serious challenge.

In 1980 an infectious disease specialist in the San Francisco Department of Public Health noticed an increase in the number of cases of amoebic dysentery, as many cases a week as had been normal for a year. A Los Angeles doctor discovered that a young gay patient, suffering from pneumocystis pneumonia, had no T helper cells. The results were so startling that the doctors ran the blood test twice. In early 1981, a New York doctor learned of six cases of Kaposi's sarcoma, all in gay men. Then a Haitian man living in New York came down with pneumocystis pneumonia, while a hospital in Queens, New York, was treating multiple cases of pneumocystis in intravenous drug users. Later in the spring, the first case of Kaposi's sarcoma occurred in San Francisco. More cases of pneumocystis were being diagnosed in Los Angeles. These signals were confusing: lots of data, but no discernable pattern.[27]

We now know that HIV targets the body's defense, attacking T helper cells, which are essential immune cells that recognize and start the body's defense against microbes. Without T cells—or with a low T-cell count—the body's immune system cannot defend itself. A person develops flu-like symptoms within two to four weeks of being infected by HIV. Then, even as the virus is laying siege to the body's immune cells, the infected person shows no symptoms and seems healthy.

For a while, the disease hides in plain sight. Eventually, though, the disease becomes symptomatic. The patient may develop fever, fatigue, thrush, diarrhea, weight loss, even pneumonia. When the level of T helper cells drops sufficiently, the patient is said to have developed acquired immune deficiency syndrome (AIDS). HIV/AIDS is slow moving. As the disease attacks the immune system over a period of years, the body succumbs to various opportunistic diseases. In the early 1980s, this was suddenly happening in New York, San Francisco, and Los Angeles. It had also been happening earlier in central Africa and Haiti, though no one had identified a pattern in the infections.

News of New York's pneumonia cases reached the CDC. At this point, the CDC believed the new disease to be associated primarily with gay men, but when one of its investigators, Mary Guinan, met with the drug users, they insisted that they did not have sex with other men. Years of experience doing contact tracing with syphilis patients had taught Guinan when to believe patients. She became convinced that the infection path for drug users was different from that for gay men. Back at the CDC, Bill Darrow, a sociologist who had done syphilis contact tracing, realized that—whatever was happening with the drug users— the disease was also sexually transmitted.[28]

Without a test for the disease, doctors had to rely on symptoms for diagnosis. On that basis, in 1983, CDC issued an advisory that gay men, intravenous (IV) drug users, hemophiliacs, and recent Haitian immigrants were high-risk groups for contracting HIV. Virus transmission could happen sexually and through blood, explaining why gay men, IV drug users, and hemophiliacs (who received frequent blood transfusions) would be in high-risk groups. DNA studies later explained the mystery of the recent Haitian immigrants: HIV had been present in Haiti for several years before its arrival in the United States. The fact that those early sufferers from HIV/AIDS—gay men, IV drug users, hemophiliacs, and Haitian immigrants—were stigmatized groups contributed to the low attention the US government paid to the disease in the early 1980s.[29]

Contact tracing for HIV/AIDS couldn't begin until 1985, after the development of a test for HIV infection. But in 1985 there was no cure for HIV/AIDS; there was only prevention. Studies had shown that HIV patients were among the most sexually active members of the population, and public health authorities knew that the disease could be transmitted through sexual contact. So, while contact tracers couldn't arrange treatment, they could still save lives by urging patients and their contacts to adopt behavioral changes.[30]

John Potterat, who directed the STD/AIDS state programs in Colorado Springs remembered, "We gave a menu of choices, like NO anal intercourse, especially of the receptive kind; or no UNPROTECTED anal intercourse ('if you're into sports, you need to suit up')"—meaning that contacts should use condoms. He added, "For IV drug users, we did something virtually identical, but emphasized not sharing needles, syringes, cookers, cottons, etc. We went into great detail . . . and told them where they could get needles, no questions asked."[31]

To prevent a disease's spread, you have to keep new infections from reaching healthy people. In other words, you want patients and their contacts to isolate. Because diseases propagate differently, isolating means taking different actions for different diseases. In the case of typhoid, which is spread through contaminated water and food, isolation means that the infected person should not prepare food or water for others. For HIV, isolation means keeping certain body fluids—blood; semen; pre-seminal, rectal, and vaginal fluids; and breast milk—away from other people. Testing blood donations, never sharing needles, reducing the number of sexual partners, and using condoms provide that kind of isolation.

In the early days of HIV, confidentiality was critical. The knowledge that someone was infected could cause them to lose their job, their livelihood, and their health insurance. The contact tracers assured people that they'd keep their HIV status confidential, and they meant it. "We can contact people without revealing who gave their name and locating information," Potterat explained to me.[32]

Positive test results meant that state or local public health authorities would be informed; a doctor who ordered an HIV test would be informed as well (as might the insurance company). This had (and has) consequences. Beginning in 1986, many states passed partner-notification laws for HIV/AIDS patients. In some states, if you do not inform a partner prior to sex that you are HIV positive, you face criminal penalties—and states have put people in jail for this.[33]

Because of the way HIV spread, the contact-tracing questions were even more intrusive than usual. Ryane Sickels, who worked as an HIV/AIDS Disease Intervention Specialist (the new form of PHA) between 2013 and 2017, described a typical conversation. It would start with the usual ways to put a person at ease, "My name is Ryane . . . I'm here because you may have been exposed to HIV. Do you have a moment? I want to see how you can benefit from other services. Everything is extremely confidential." The discussion would quickly move into more probing questions: "I want to talk about actual behavior. When was the last time you had sex with a man? What type of sex was it? Was it anal? Oral? When was the last time you had sex with a woman? Anal? Oral? Vaginal? Do your partners have sex with other people? Do you know your partner's health status? Has your partner ever been tested?"[34]

Only then would Ryane turn to partner notification, "Do you have primary partners? Secondary partners? Any anonymous partners? Who are these partners?" Ryane would ask for contact information and remind the patient that the conversation was entirely confidential. She emphasized patient confidentiality, for it was the most important message she had to convey. "I want to see you benefit from other services," she would say, "Here's my card. I'm going to follow up with you in a few days."[35]

Then Ryane would reach out to each of the person's contacts to tell them they had been exposed to HIV and should get tested. She would tell them that they'd been exposed, but not by whom. A contact tracer is responsible for protecting public health, but they must respect and honor a patient's confidentiality and autonomy. Their role cannot work without that—after all, people are sharing their information voluntarily.[36]

In the first half-dozen years of the HIV/AIDS epidemic, over two-thirds of infected patients in the United States were gay; IV drug users were the second largest cohort. Contact tracing was not made easier by the fact that the Public Health Services didn't have any (openly) gay contact tracers. The PHAs had started out white and male; in the 1950s, some Black employees were hired. Women were not added to the pool until 1970. And until the AIDS crisis made the need critically clear, the agency had not made a deliberate effort to hire gay and lesbian contact tracers. Even so, and despite the fact that trans and nonbinary people were both a significant part of the LGBTQ community and experienced high rates of HIV infections, they weren't hired as contact tracers until decades later.[37]

Over time, the demographics of the HIV/AIDS population in the United States has changed. A disease once associated with (white) gay men, intravenous drug users, hemophiliacs, and Haitian immigrants now primarily affects racial and ethnic minorities. Black Americans make up 13 percent of the US population, but 42 percent of people in the United States with HIV/AIDS. Similarly, 18 percent of the US population identifies as Latinx (of any race), but 27 percent of people in the United States with HIV/AIDS are Latinx.[38]

The CDC has long believed in contact tracers and epidemiologists working together. The two groups hold different skills and speak different languages; contact tracers provide expertise in patient interviewing and education, while epidemiologists ask the scientific questions that uncover the dynamics of a disease's spread. Asking "Whom do you sleep with?" might help a contact tracer find the next infected person. But understanding what the connections were within a social network—and then connecting with key players—could allow a contact tracer to stop an infection from spreading through the group.[39]

Even when compared with other pandemic diseases, Ebola stands out as terrifying. The disease kills up to 80 percent of those infected, with death following in a matter of days after exposure. Ebola's symptoms are frightening. They start with intense fatigue, loss of appetite, headaches, muscle and joint pain, nausea, vomiting, diarrhea, and, oddly, hiccups; the final stages can include seizures, internal and external bleeding, and shock. The disease is caused by five different, closely related, viruses; four affect humans with levels of virulence ranging from 40 to 90 percent. The virus is easily spread via body fluids (both from the living and the dead), putting family members and medical professionals alike at great risk.[40]

There is no cure for Ebola, although some recent drugs seem promising. Treatment addresses the symptoms: hydration for loss of fluids (either oral or intravenously) and medication for stopping pain, fever, and diarrhea. The earlier a patient arrives at a treatment center, the more likely they are to survive.[41]

Ebola first emerged in near simultaneous outbreaks in Sudan and Zaire (now the Democratic Republic of Congo) in 1976. It has appeared multiple times since then, largely in East and Central Africa. Most outbreaks have been relatively small, involving several hundred people, but the 2014–2016 outbreak in West Africa—in Guinea, Sierra Leone, and Liberia—infected 29,000 people, of whom 11,000 died.[42]

The earlier outbreaks in East and Central Africa were identified within two months, but it took three months before public health authorities recognized the Ebola outbreak in West Africa. This was another case of a disease appearing in an unexpected place, looking like something else (perhaps cholera, or malaria). The lagging realization that Ebola had appeared in West Africa enabled the disease to spread and contributed to the outbreak's severity. The spread was exacerbated by the epidemic's start in a dense, highly mobile population center at the border of three nations.[43]

Consider the situation in Liberia, where people already distrusted the government as a result of over a decade of civil wars that had only ended in 2003. The government's early actions increased the public's distrust and created resistance to public health orders. Quarantine orders such as the one that locked in a poor and densely packed neighborhood in Monrovia failed to provide sufficient food and water for residents—and so the orders were disobeyed.[44]

The Liberian government's approach to treating the ill also frightened the public. Infected people were taken to Ebola Treatment Units, but during the worst of the epidemic, when the facilities couldn't cope with the influx of patients, families were not informed of a relative's death or survival. The centers were seen as death camps, which meant that people who needed help stayed away. The policies were designed for speed because, as one public health official put it, in a medical crisis like Ebola, "If you go slow at the beginning . . . you can very rapidly start a brushfire that turns into a major disaster."[45]

Government burial policy made everything worse. In West Africa it is traditional for family, and sometimes friends, to wash and clean the body of the deceased. But because contact with the body fluids of an Ebola patient can spread the disease, the government prohibited burial ceremonies. A safe burial for a person who has died of Ebola requires that the body be handled only by people fully suited up in protective gear, with the corpse buried in a sealed body bag. Nevertheless, people continued to perform burial rituals on loved ones who had died at home, further spreading the disease.[46]

The public's distrust meant the government's policies weren't being followed. Soon, the medical situation in Liberia had spun out of control. With Ebola's high transmission and death rates, this appeared to be an insurmountable disaster. Contact tracing was the natural solution, but WHO officials resisted the approach. Teams working in the urban areas didn't believe contact tracing would work—and epidemiologists modeling different interventions hadn't been able to put a measure on how community involvement might benefit contact tracing.[47]

But health workers tried contact tracing nevertheless—and it changed the whole picture. I spoke with three Liberians who explained how that happened. Lassana Jabateh, a community health director, and Garmai Cyrus and Willis Archie Yasnine, both mental health counselors, all work for Partners in Health, an international organization focusing on community-based public health interventions.

Cyrus said that, in the early days of the outbreak, people encountered a lot of misinformation about the disease. Some believed government officials had manufactured the disease and were trying to spread it; others simply distrusted the government and so rejected the control measures, including travel bans and safe burials. The government's comments didn't help. "Politicians and lawmakers didn't believe in Ebola," said Cyrus. "They politicized the situation, terming the president as planning war and that it was a plan to get at the opposition. Communities became resistant to the reality of Ebola," she explained.[48]

"We had to change community perception on what was Ebola," said Yasnine. Bringing in trusted community leaders— elders, town chiefs, commissioners, zone (village) heads, religious leaders, teachers, and the secret societies, culturally important groups that pass on traditional values between generations within the communities—was key to educating the community about Ebola and convincing residents to protect themselves. It also enabled contact tracing. "Community leaders can tell us who might be a contact tracer," said Yasnine. "There was lots of community engagement [in picking the contact tracers]," Jabateh added.[49]

Engaging community leaders meant that contact tracers could identify and isolate cases and quarantine their contacts. "As a family stayed home to isolate themselves, the community organized to get the water for drinking and bathing. And the community went to the market to buy food for the family. Partners in Health paid," noted Cyrus.[50]

Jabateh and Yasnine explained that if a community had fifty houses, they'd recruit twenty-five contact tracers. Each house typically has three to four households, so a contact tracer would be responsible for keeping track of about six to eight families, or around forty people. During Ebola, the contact tracer's role was to check in daily with everyone, find out if anyone was ill or showing any kind of symptoms, and, if so, report it. The person would be taken to holding centers or the Ebola Treatment Units, where they'd be tested. It's a different model for contact tracing than the United States used for syphilis or HIV/AIDS, but it's a model that worked.

With the involvement of community leaders, the Ebola outbreak turned around. Contact tracing was crucial to that outcome. And contact tracing can only work when there is trust.

Trust was also key to South Korea's early response to COVID-19. But before South Korea got a pandemic response right, the country had gotten one badly wrong. Middle East respiratory syndrome (MERS) first appeared in Saudi Arabia in 2012. A zoonotic disease that spread from camels, MERS's human-to-human transmission is low, with R_0 below 1. But it's MERS's high fatality rate that makes it so dangerous. Of the 1,100 people known to be infected by MERS by the end of 2015, 470 had died.[51]

The index case in South Korea was a sixty-eight-year-old man who had traveled to the Middle East. A week after his return, the patient had become ill and went "doctor shopping," visiting four different hospitals over a ten-day period. By the time he was diagnosed, the index patient had infected twenty-eight other people, two of whom infected 109 more. A total of 185 people were infected with MERS in South Korea in 2015, and all but two of them acquired the disease in a hospital. The system had failed spectacularly. It failed to diagnose a key case, failed to quarantine the "superspreaders," allowed caregiver visits in the face of a highly contagious disease, and mismanaged hospital infections. The biggest spread had occurred from the superspreaders who visited multiple health care facilities in search of help.[52]

With COVID-19, South Korea was determined not to repeat its failure to manage MERS. The public health authorities knew that halting an epidemic meant test, isolate, trace, and treat. Post MERS, the country put in place policies designed to remove barriers to contact tracing during an epidemic. When COVID-19 arrived, South Korea was ready with simplified approval rules for diagnostic tests and exceptions to its data privacy law.[53]

The first case of COVID-19 in Korea was confirmed on January 20, 2020. Within five weeks, South Korea was able to perform 15,000 diagnostic tests per day. The United States, which had its first confirmed case the same day as South Korea, only caught up to that testing rate a month later.[54]

Aided by digital data, contact tracing also happened quickly. Under the Infectious Disease Prevention and Control Act, which was passed after MERS, the Ministry of Health and Welfare and the Korean Centers for Disease Control and Prevention could collect and share cellular phone location data, immigration records, medical and prescription records, closed circuit television footage (CCTV), records of credit card transactions, and transit pass records for infected people and people suspected of being infected. The location information is quite detailed, listing 10,000 locations for a single individual in a two-week period, for example.[55]

South Korean contact tracers examined CCTV records to determine who was likely to have become infected by a contagious individual. Was the infected person at the ATM wearing a mask? If so, the shortness of the encounter plus the mask meant that anyone in the immediate vicinity was probably safe and therefore didn't need to be traced. Did they eat at a restaurant? That constitutes a long exposure—and, of course, without a mask. The contact tracers would study the CCTV: were other patrons nearby? By obtaining credit card records for the time in question, the contact tracers could locate other patrons who'd potentially been exposed. They would be put under self-quarantine for fourteen days (the incubation period for SARS-CoV-2).[56]

In South Korea, quarantine violation carries a fine of up to KRW10 million (approximately $8,300) and a year's imprisonment. Quarantine is enforced: the exposed person must use a "safety-protection app" to report their symptoms twice daily. The app also lets the government monitor the person's location. If an exposed person exhibits symptoms, they get tested. Test, trace, isolate.[57]

South Korea made it easy to get tested. By mid-March, the country had established 600 test centers. To avoid a repeat of the MERS situation, in which spread occurred inside hospitals, South Korea built stand-alone "phone booth" testing sites. The booths take one person at a time. The tester is on the outside, and negative air pressure prevents virus particles from escaping. The booths are disinfected and ventilated between tests, which takes seven minutes. Results were available within two days.[58]

Anyone testing positive with mild symptoms was sent to a treatment support center, while those with moderate to severe symptoms were hospitalized. The government also provided emergency disaster relief for anyone suffering from COVID-19—easing the financial burden of self-quarantining.[59]

South Korea's efforts were successful. The nation had largely contained the virus when there was a sudden spike of infections in the city of Daegu in February 2020. Relatively quickly, the authorities traced the outbreak to a church service, specifically, to "Patient #31," who had attended with a fever. Worshippers at the Shincheonji Church of Jesus did not wear masks and stood close together; by the time that officials realized that the infection was spreading, the numbers were in the hundreds. But the lessons from MERS stood, and by late March, South Korea was down to double-digit numbers of new cases per day.[60]

One tool that South Korea used to prevent the virus's spread was publishing information about the movements of infected cases, including the public transport they used. Public health authorities posted this information on websites, blogs, and social media accounts. Some districts also released information on the businesses and apartment complexes—60 percent of Koreans live in large apartment buildings—that infected people had been in prior to diagnosis. This helped others figure out where they might have been exposed; this information, along with widely available testing, made it easy for residents to determine whether they might be infected. But the publicity associated with providing this information also created negative impacts. COVID-19 is not now considered a disease that spreads easily via surfaces, but South Korea's public health bulletins meant that a coffee shop that had been visited by an infected person might soon find itself without customers.[61]

The government published whether the infected people had been wearing masks and whether their homes had been disinfected, as well as information on age and gender. The bulletins did not expressly name individuals, but publishing this much information could nonetheless violate privacy. In May 2020, a twenty-nine-year-old man infected with COVID-19 went bar hopping in Itaewon, a Seoul neighborhood with bars catering to LGBTQ customers. Public bulletins listed the hot spots of a possible new outbreak without revealing who'd been at the bars. But a positive test result in the days afterwards could quickly lead friends and family to draw their own conclusions about an individual's sexual identity. In this case, contact tracing involved contacting thousands of people.[62]

The World Health Organization says that the best way to contain an epidemic is to test, trace, and isolate. That's what doctors did in Bradford, England, to quickly stop a potential epidemic. With syphilis, the PHAs could do one better: test, trace, and cure. Containing the HIV/AIDS epidemic began with test, trace, and efforts at harm reduction; later it involved treatment. The Ebola outbreaks have all been stopped with test, trace, and isolate. And South Korea's approach to test, trace, and isolate has, so far, managed to contain COVID-19 in that country.

Is South Korea's technological solution exportable? Would it be possible to implement such a plan while protecting residents' privacy? To answer that, we need a better understanding of the technological approaches.

3 ADDING TECHNOLOGY TO CONTACT TRACING

When the cook from Bradford Children's Hospital was belatedly diagnosed with smallpox, it didn't take much time to do contact tracing and determine whom he might have infected. As we've seen, contact tracing—test, trace, isolate—has been successful in ending smallpox, as well as in limiting typhoid, HIV/AIDS, Ebola, and other infectious diseases.

Notwithstanding South Korea's early success, COVID-19 presents a serious challenge to this model. The disease is elusive, often spreading from people who may not yet be showing symptoms—or who may even be asymptomatic. The infection develops and spreads quickly; a person may be not only infected but also infectious within days of exposure. Superspreading incidents, in which a large number of people become ill from exposure by a single person, have occurred multiple times. All of this increases the need for public health authorities to quickly identify an infected person's contacts. The lack of tests, partially a result of some governments' reluctance to employ them, and political and economic opposition to isolation have further impeded contact tracing.

Diseases like COVID-19 that spread through respiratory droplets, even without symptoms, require contact tracers to ask a different set of questions than diseases that involve more prolonged or intimate contact. Instead of developing an understanding of an infected person's social networks, a contact tracer wants to know, "Where were you within the last two weeks?" They also need to know the answer to a more difficult question: "Who was near you?" Sometimes these people's identities might be known to you, and sometimes not. Chance encounters at the convenience store or in a coffee shop take on outsized importance.[1]

The information that contact tracers need to track the spread of the coronavirus is information that a smartphone—the radio in your pocket—can collect. Smartphones offer the capability to reveal not just where you've been, but who's been near you. In theory, smartphones can inform anonymous strangers on the subway or at the movie theater that they were exposed to someone infected with COVID-19. You might not have exchanged a single word—or perhaps even noticed each other. This kind of capability could be important wherever large numbers of people gather closely together: a factory floor, a church service, a nightclub, a large lecture hall. Let's take a look at how this idea might play out in practice.[2]

With the pandemic spreading across international borders in early 2020, some governments thought they might be able to contain it by tracking infected people and isolating them and their contacts—even without testing. South Korea, as we have seen, used cell tower locations and other types of digital data in combination with a heavy dose of contact tracers to track both known and unknown contacts of infected persons. Israel similarly attempted to contain the virus with a cell tower–based surveillance tool employed by Shin Bet, the Israeli internal intelligence service, for tracking terrorists. Could this approach to location tracking work?

Cell towers provide a very rough measure of location, perhaps useful for tracking bank robbers or terrorists, but less so for tracking respiratory infections. We know more now about how the coronavirus spreads than we did in early 2020, but even then, it was clear that the virus spread largely through close contacts. The CDC suggested we should be concerned about interactions closer than "six feet." More specifically, someone is a "close contact" of an infected person if they've been within six feet for at least fifteen minutes during the person's most infectious period, defined as the span between two days before symptoms appear and when the patient began to isolate. For asymptomatic carriers, the infectious period is unclear; for the purposes of contact tracing, it has been defined as the period starting two days before testing and lasting through the beginning of isolation.[3]

The Israeli tool collected locations at nowhere near this level of specificity, tracking only the cell towers from which calls and texts were made and received. The tool reported people as being in close proximity even when they were separated by many feet, often with a closed door, wall, or window between them.[4]

On its own, then, cell tower location doesn't provide sufficient accuracy to determine who might have been exposed to the coronavirus. But signal strength from multiple nearby towers can provide greater accuracy as to where a phone—and a person—is located. In South Korea, contact tracers combined cell tower location with additional data to accurately pinpoint the actual locations of infected people. For example, "On Saturday October 10, 2020, patient 5703 went to the Hannam-dong cultural facilities from 6:16–6:18 pm, stopped into the Hannam-dong cafe from 6:24–6:46 pm, returned to the cultural center at 6:52 and stayed til 9:38, then stopped at the Hannam-dong convenience store from 9:38–9:42 pm."[5]

A smartphone's GPS signals provide finer precision, with GPS-enabled smartphones typically reporting location to an accuracy of sixteen feet. But that accuracy can be affected by many factors. In cities, signals might bounce off buildings; in the country, trees. Nor do GPS signals typically penetrate into buildings—so sometimes the GPS signal will say you're inside a shop when you're actually sitting on a bench outside. GPS can say whether two people went into the same subway station, but it won't determine whether they sat in the same car.[6]

Even so, GPS signals have been useful in other ways during the COVID-19 pandemic. Some governments, including Kenya, Ecuador, and South Korea, are using GPS location to track individuals who have been ordered to isolate or quarantine. GPS information can also be used to track group behavior. Throughout the COVID-19 crisis, tech companies have provided aggregated information about people's movement collected from smartphone apps. In the Netherlands and the Philippines, government officials used this data to see whether people were following public health recommendations to "stay home, stay safe." Washington State drew on similar information to guide its reopening plans. But the data collection draws information only from those who use smartphones and their associated mapping services, a demographic that generally skews younger and wealthier than the population at large.[7]

While cell tower location and GPS didn't appear particularly useful for tracking close contacts, others forms of smartphone radio signals looked more promising. In addition to cell tower location and GPS signals, cell phones can collect location information using Wi-Fi networks. Each network broadcasts its base station number; the phone sweeps up all the networks it encounters, even if it never connects to any of them. Phones share that information: Androids with a Google server, iPhones with an

Apple server. The servers use a previously constructed database to look at the signal strengths and the intersection of the networks to determine where the phone is. The Wi-Fi method is not particularly precise, however, and would not typically be able to determine whether two people were in that critical six-foot proximity range.

Some Wi-Fi networks can do better. Harvard University piloted a Wi-Fi–based program, TraceFi, to see if it could usefully supplement manual contact tracing of infected people. TraceFi was based on the idea that if someone at Harvard tests positive for the coronavirus, in some cases university IT staff could use Wi-Fi signals to determine where that person was during their contagious period. Such information can jog the patient's memory about who else might have been nearby. To find their users' locations—that lobby, this classroom—Harvard relied on registration information users supply when they sign onto the Harvard Wi-Fi network. The two-month test project showed proof of concept, but not efficacy, and was ended in September 2020.[8]

Bluetooth, which was designed to connect small, low-power devices—for instance, to connect your wireless mouse with your desktop computer, or your phone to another to enable hot spots—is a more promising tool for identifying proximity. An even better option than Bluetooth is Bluetooth Low Energy (BLE), a variant of Bluetooth used for transmitting small amounts of data. BLE is used for such functions as streaming music to your headphones or transmitting your smart thermometer reading to your phone.

Now imagine an app that broadcasts a phone's presence using BLE technology. Any phone in the immediate vicinity running the same app would pick up the signal. That such radio signals attenuate—weaken—as the distance grows is a decided advantage of BLE for testing proximity. The stronger the signal, the more likely the two people were close by.

If both phones were broadcasting the signal, each would receive notice of the other's proximity. This would be extraordinarily useful information if one of the phone's owners were later discovered to have been infected with COVID-19 at the time the phones—and their owners—were near each other. The phones could exchange this information even if their owners were strangers, for example, if they were just sitting next to each other on a train or in a movie theater.

With this understanding of the various ways that phones signal their locations, let's look more closely at the first generation of contact-tracing apps.

Singapore's TraceTogether was the first COVID-19 app that emphasized proximity—"Who's been nearby the last two weeks?"—over location—"Where have you been?" Launched in mid-March 2020, the app uses BLE technology to exchange proximity information with nearby BLE-enabled devices.

When users sign up for TraceTogether, they provide their phone number and their "unique identification number"—a government ID used for a wide range of activities. This is a government-owned app; by signing up, users are authorizing the government to view essentially all the information that phones collect from the app. The Ministry of Health (MOH) creates identifiers that each phone sends out via BLE. These identifiers are strings based on the user's phone number. To protect users' privacy, these identifiers change frequently, so the app also keeps track of the time window for each identifier. An MOH server downloads twenty-four hours' worth of new identifiers to Trace-Together users daily.[9]

When two users of the app, say, Alyssa and Ben, are in close proximity, their phones receive and store each other's identifiers. If Ben were to later test positive for COVID-19, one of the first things an MOH contact tracer would ask him is whether he's been using TraceTogether. If so, MOH will upload information from Ben's phone: the exchanged identifiers of people who were also using TraceTogether and whom Ben encountered over the previous twenty-five days. The health ministry may also upload location information from other apps on Ben's phone.[10]

Because Alyssa was near Ben at some point during his infectious period, one of her identifiers ends up at the MOH, which can then decipher it as belonging to Alyssa. But MOH doesn't call Alyssa right away; nor does Alyssa receive an automated message from the app. Not every identifier on Ben's phone is linked to a close contact in serious risk of contracting COVID-19. If Ben had been using public transportation at popular hours, or going out to bars or restaurants, his phone may have stored thousands of identifiers. Contacting everyone associated with each of these and asking them to isolate for fourteen days from the time of exposure is simply not plausible. The contact tracer needs to do some investigating.[11]

An MOH contact tracer talks with Ben to discover where he had been and what he'd been doing. Ben's singing with other people while infectious carries great risk of spread; his listening quietly to a lecture does not. The contact tracer combines information on Ben's activities with the exposure information uploaded from the phone to determine which people who were exposed to Ben are most at risk of contracting COVID-19. Then, and only then, does the MOH start calling some of Ben's contacts. MOH also obtains the exchanged identifiers on the contact's phone so that it can repeat the process if the contact tests positive.[12]

This is how TraceTogether works in theory, but not everything functioned according to plan. One problem involved operating system incompatibility. Apple's iPhones use a proprietary format for BLE communications for apps running in background mode—that is, when the smartphone is actively using another app. When that occurs, an iPhone can't send to or receive BLE notifications from Android phones, and vice versa. Health authorities in Singapore recommended that iPhone TraceTogether users keep the app actively running (in the foreground) in situations with high risk of exposure, for instance, when riding a bus or a train during rush hour. When active, the app would revert to using a communications format that both Androids and iPhones used, thereby solving the problem. But users found that continuously running the app in foreground rapidly drained the battery. It's also disruptive; commuting time is exactly when phone users want to play games, read e-books or do anything but just run the app. Later the TraceTogether team figured out a way to have iPhones run the apps in background and yet send and receive BLE notifications with Android phones—but not with other iPhones.[13]

At first, use of TraceTogether was fully voluntary. In April 2020, however, Singapore experienced an outbreak of COVID-19, with the number of cases spiraling from around 1,000 early in the month to over 26,000 six weeks later. The outbreak occurred in dormitories housing migrant workers, who make up one-third of Singapore's workforce. The Singaporean government now requires migrant workers living in such dormitories or working in the nation's crucial construction, marine, or petrochemical sectors to use the app. Many workplaces also require employees to use the app as a precondition for work.[14]

Singapore's TraceTogether app constitutes *decentralized* collection of proximity information and *centralized* use of that information. Until Ben is diagnosed with COVID-19 and contacted by the MOH, Alyssa's identifiers remain only on Ben's phone. It is, in that sense, decentralized. But once Ben has been contacted by MOH, he must upload the proximity identifiers his phone has collected to an MOH server. That's centralized use, and it means that the Singapore government learns who's been around Ben over the previous three weeks—even those unlikely to be at risk of contracting COVID-19.

The success of TraceTogether—and all proximity-based apps—depends on the rate of adoption. If Alyssa and Ben are both on a bus but Ben isn't using the app, TraceTogether can't record Alyssa's exposure. If only 10 percent of the population were using TraceTogether, assuming infectious people were randomly distributed, that 10 percent would find 10 percent of exposures—or TraceTogether would have a 1 percent chance of reporting that Alyssa was actually exposed (10 percent × 10 percent). If, on the other hand, 56 percent of the population were using the app, then it would catch 31 percent of exposures. A study from the University of Oxford suggests that this level of adoption might be enough to suppress the disease's spread. Singapore's experience shows that convincing people to use such apps is not easy: by July 2020, only 35 percent of Singaporeans had downloaded TraceTogether (and many of them did so because the government required them to).[15]

With adoption rates low, Singapore tried a different approach. The government distributed small devices—dongles—for free. These were to be worn whenever people went outside or anticipated being near people outside their household. The dongles only collected proximity information. If someone tested positive for COVID-19, public health officials would collect their device and download their proximity history for the previous twenty-five days. The first distribution of 10,000 devices went to elderly people who hadn't been able to use TraceTogether because they lacked smartphones.[16]

TraceTogether was only part of Singapore's approach to contact tracing; another was SafeEntry, a digital check-in system introduced in May 2020. Anyone entering a somewhat public place—a taxi, supermarket, large retail outlet, mall, bank, hotel, library, museum, movie theater, or other public building—must provide their name, national ID, and phone number through an automated system that feeds the data to the MOH for contact-tracing purposes. Though potentially effective in tracing the spread of an outbreak, this approach creates a world with essentially no anonymity.[17]

In India, the Aarogya Setu app—Hindi for "the bridge for liberation from disease"—had 127 million downloads by mid-July 2020, less than four months after its introduction. India has been racing into automated tools for all aspects of modern life. The country's biometric national identity system, Aadhaar, uses biometric identifiers—iris scans, fingerprints, and photos—to provide Indian citizens with unique twelve-digit numbers.

Almost all of India's 1.3 billion people are enrolled in Aadhaar. Officials intended the ID system to regulate access to such government benefits as rice rations, but it quickly became embedded throughout Indian life. Before the Indian Supreme Court ruled against the practice in 2018, banks and insurance companies demanded registration with the Aadhaar card as a condition of service. Schools required students to have it to access lunch, and some temples required it as a condition for participating in religious rituals. Aadhaar's introduction was, as one privacy scholar described it, an example of "technology before policy."[18]

With Aarogya Setu, a government app, India seems to be on a similar path of developing a technological solution to a problem without first determining the policies governing its use. The contact-tracing app combines three apps in one package. The first collects users' symptoms and provides an assessment of a person's risk of COVID-19; the second informs the public about COVID-19 hot spots and predicts where new outbreaks might occur; the third does proximity checking.

Aarogya Setu takes a Silicon Valley approach to providing services: collect lots of data and automate responses. Maybe that's no surprise; it's being run under the Ministry of Electronics and Information Technology (MeitY) rather than the Ministry of Health and Family Welfare. When users register, they provide their name, phone number, age, sex, and countries visited in the last thirty days—and also agree to Bluetooth proximity checking and GPS tracking. Aarogya Setu then asks the user to do a simple self-assessment, answering a few questions about symptoms (cough, fever, difficulty breathing), abbreviated medical history (any history of diabetes, hypertension, lung or heart disease), international travel in the previous fourteen days, and two factors that increase a person's risk of having contracted the disease: interactions with or living with someone who has recently tested positive or being a health care worker who examined infected patients without wearing protective gear.[19]

The app provides an automated assessment of the person's risk of being infected and makes recommendations regarding isolation and the need to get tested. The value of this is unclear. The government does not enforce isolation, and, even six months into the pandemic, testing continues to lag. There's also a failure of follow-up. By mid-summer 2020, the country was overwhelmed with COVID-19 cases. In many places, it was simply not possible for contact tracers to follow up with known cases.[20]

The information collected by the app can be used in other ways, too. In a podcast interview shortly after the app launched,

Lalitesh Katragadda, who heads the product and architecture teams at Aarogya Setu, said that as disease hot spots are emerging, the information the app has collected "will allow us to control and trace people and quarantine people early, and contain [COVID-19] much faster than we would otherwise." Within weeks of the app's launch, the government reported that Aarogya Setu anticipated identifying over 1,200 emerging COVID-19 "hot spots" that might not have been found otherwise. But this didn't appear to be the case. Raman Jit Singh Chima, Senior International Counsel and Asia Pacific Policy Director of Access Now, a civil society group, told me: "When Aarogya Setu took hot spots to the states, the states said, 'We already had that data.'" He added later, "As summer progressed, it became clear that the state government responses to COVID-19 spikes and public health responses to contain the rise were not primarily relying on Aarogya Setu and its data, insights."[21]

Aarogya Setu also lets users know the number of COVID-19 cases within a 0.5-, 1-, 2-, 5-, and 10-kilometer radius, the idea being to warn a user about the risk of traveling in certain areas (5–10 kilometers is the maximum distance that urban commuters tend to travel), but it is its third capability, proximity tracing, that has garnered the most attention. This function works across three different operating systems: Android, iOS (Apple), and KaiOS (a system used in inexpensive smartphones that have become popular in India since 2018).[22]

When Aadya and Bhargav encounter each other while using Aarogya Setu, their devices conduct a Bluetooth proximity exchange. In contrast to TraceTogether and almost all other proximity-checking apps, Aarogya Setu does not use temporary IDs for its users. Instead, the app uses a static identifier for each user, which allows a snooper—someone collecting the BLE notifications—to track app users' locations. Anyone from criminals to governments could learn a person's exact location simply by tracking their BLE signals. The Indian Army especially objected to this feature, ordering its personnel not to use Aarogya Setu while in the office, during military operations, or at any sensitive location.[23]

If neither Aadya nor Bhargav tests positive for COVID-19, the record of their encounter—they exchange temporary identifiers—never leaves their phones. But if Bhargav later tests positive for COVID-19, data covering his encounters with others and thirty days' worth of his location history are uploaded to a government server. At that point, the app calculates Aadya's risk of exposure and passes the information on to the Ministry of Health or the state health department contact tracers. Aadya may receive an exposure notification from the app that she is at a low risk of infection (encouraging her to be cautious), or she may receive a call from a contact tracer if the risk is moderate or high. If the latter, she may be told to isolate and also reminded to dismiss her maid—the assumption being that anyone who owns a smartphone also employs domestic workers. Aarogya Setu, like TraceTogether, retains a role for public health workers as essential players in successful contact tracing—when there are contact tracers available to make those calls.[24]

In early May, the Indian government made Aarogya Setu compulsory for all public and private-sector employees—that is, all workers in the formal economy—as well as for anyone living in a containment zone (areas that have been isolated due to COVID-19 cases). That order was rescinded just two weeks later. Some Indian states required that all travelers use Aarogya Setu before boarding a train or plane; that order, too, was later rescinded. Some shopping malls, food markets, and government offices have turned away people for not running the app. Several months later, the government settled on "strongly encouraging" the app's use. In August, the developers provided an interface for companies to query the app about their employee's health status.[25]

When it comes to telecommunications, India is two countries. In the cities, smartphone use is high. In contrast, rural Indians frequently have "feature phones" that can access email, GPS, and some social networks, but lack the BLE capability required for proximity tracing. For feature phones, Aarogya Setu includes the assessment test, which provides the government with information about possible spread of the disease, but feature phone users don't receive the benefits of contact tracing and exposure notification capabilities to which the 40 percent of India's population with smartphones have access. To the extent that the app diverts resources from the poorer three-fifths of India's population, the app may be causing more harm than good.[26]

Given India's inability to manage the three legs of the contact-tracing stool—test, trace, and isolate—the government's hard push for residents to adopt Aarogya Setu may seem surprising. It appears to be related to the "National Health Stack," a digitized health care repository due to come online in 2022. A project with a big vision intended to simplify access to health records, streamline billing, and control medical costs through an efficient supply of drugs and medical supplies, the National Health Stack is premised on easier access to data, lots of data. An Aadhaar number will be the identity of choice. It's notable that privacy doesn't come up until two-thirds of the way through the government's strategy document describing the National Health Stack.[27]

Katragadda said that some of Aarogya Setu's data will be automatically transferred to the National Health Stack. He assured me that only results of diagnostic tests and related information would be transferred—and only at the explicit request of the patient. That claim, however, doesn't stand up to scrutiny. As of this writing, the only document governing the use of data in Aarogya Setu is a "protocol" issued by MeitY. The protocol specifies which agencies may receive the information (largely, but not solely, those involved with health care) and the length of time that these data may be retained. But an analysis by one of India's civil society organizations, the Internet Freedom Foundation (IFF), found the policy fell far short of protecting privacy. Of greatest concern was how the policy allowed the government to share information about close contacts and location for anything from contact tracing to medical research to managing the pandemic. IFF also noted there was no policy for deleting contact, location, and the self-assessment test if the user requests it—and no explanation of whether limits on data retention apply to so-called anonymized data."[28]

By July 2020, three months after its introduction, Aarogya Setu's downloads were declining even while the number of COVID-19 cases in India was soaring. But with so many businesses pushing customers and employees to use the app, Aarogya Setu continued to collect patient health data.

Let's take a step back and think about what happens when a person uses these apps. When Ben and Alyssa's phones exchange proximity information while using TraceTogether, no one learns about anything unless Ben tests positive for COVID-19. Then a government contact tracer receives information about their encounters. The phone collects records of two types of meetings: those Ben knows about and may recall—whether it was something that happened while sitting next to someone indoors or a less risky outside encounter—as well as the anonymous ones Ben is less likely to remember, for instance, how long he stood next to a given person on a bus or in a department store. Based on a conversation with Ben and data from the phone, the contact tracer assesses whether Alyssa was a "close contact."

If she is, Alyssa will be told to quarantine. That means no going to work, no food shopping, no taking care of her children or other relatives. It's restrictive and hard. In a nation where there's no unemployment benefits unless you're a citizen or permanent resident—and 30 percent of workers in Singapore are not—the consequences can be severe. And all of this is solely on the basis of an estimate of whether Alyssa is likely to become infected—an estimate because the app and contact tracer cannot know for sure.

If Alyssa later turns out to be infected as a result of her encounter with Ben, the quarantine order was a wise choice. If not, it was a costly one, with Alyssa bearing the expense. Either way, the decision was out of her hands; once the app noted the encounter and Ben was diagnosed, MOH determined Alyssa's need to quarantine.

The situation in India is slightly different. If Bhargav tests positive and is using Aarogya Setu, Aadya may be called by a contact tracer and told to isolate. As of this writing, enforcement has not been as strong as in Singapore—and so Aadya may experience no adverse consequences when the public health agency learns of her exposure. That could change, of course.

Using TraceTogether or Aarogya Setu means that if either Ben or Bhargav become ill with COVID-19, their Ministries of Health receive information on their phone about their encounters. Both Singapore and India have instituted policies that say this information is only to be used for health purposes related to the pandemic. But if there's one certainty about data collection, it's "function creep": the increase in uses of collected information. Without even a parliamentary discussion—let alone a vote—Israel repurposed a secret database of cellphone location information used for terrorist investigations for use in COVID-19 contact tracing. The country used the database to enforce quarantine on close contacts of infected people. Function creep happens everywhere. US criminal wiretap law, for instance, started out limiting the use of wiretap warrants to twenty-five different types of "serious" crimes; now that list numbers nearly 100.[29]

In this situation, extending a government's ability to collect location and proximity information on the people within its borders poses a serious threat to civil liberties. Contact tracing surveils and contains infected people and their contacts in the name of public health, but contact-tracing apps could potentially surveil everyone—especially if the apps are widely used. As epidemiologists and computer scientists began thinking about using that radio in your pocket to aid contact tracing, the privacy issue lay dead center in front of them.

4 PROTECTING PRIVACY WHILE TRACING DISEASE

Contact tracers invade the privacy of infected individuals in order to protect the public's health. To the extent that it is possible, providing confidentiality is critical to the success of their endeavor. During the height of the HIV/AIDS epidemic, those infected were barred from schools, fired from jobs, and refused medical treatment by frightened health care providers—even though the actual chances of transmitting the disease in those situations was low. While contact tracers inevitably share some portion of what they learn with their local public health authorities, they can and do keep a patient's information confidential within the constraints of broader public safety.[1]

To do their work properly, a contact tracer needs to learn whom you might have exposed while infectious. For typhoid, the answer to that question might be the people you had cooked for; for syphilis and HIV/AIDS, it might be people with whom you had sex or shared needles. For COVID-19, the answer depends on where you've been, who's been near you, and what you were doing while you were there. Such information may seem, at first glance, less invasive than the question of whom you're sleeping with. But the identification of the places you've been and the people you've been with, let alone what you were doing with them, says a lot about you.

A trip to a gynecologist's office followed by a stop at a maternity shop tells one story. But if those are followed a few weeks later by a late-night visit to a hospital emergency room and no more trips to the gynecologist, this reveals a different tale, one that even the woman's closest friends might not know about. Phone GPS data can disclose that a person stayed out past a government-imposed curfew, or that someone with a history of drug-related arrests stayed over at his aunt's, putting her at risk of losing her public housing apartment.[2]

It's easy to identify people just from their location data; a rough sense of where people are during the workday and at night is enough to identify 95 percent of people. Patterns of location information can reveal an extraordinary amount about a person's habits and history. If you stop by a church for Alcoholics Anonymous on Tuesdays, Thursdays, and Saturdays at 7, your regular appearance at the church at those hours, combined with the fact that you're not religious, might disclose your attempt to recover from a drinking problem. If you hang out in a particular neighborhood on Friday and Saturday nights, that might give away that you're gay.[3]

Proximity data can similarly reveal activities you might not want to share. Possibly you ran into an old girlfriend on the subway and the two of you stopped for a coffee, an encounter you'd just as soon not mention at home. Maybe some of your friends work for the competition, and while you're careful not to discuss proprietary information when you meet, your weekly get-togethers could cause trouble for you with your boss. Or you're a journalist; a list of who you're meeting with might endanger your sources.

Your social network can reveal your politics or sexual preferences. Public knowledge of whom you spend time with can put you at risk of social, political, and legal consequences. Maybe you spend time with a group of old friends whose political views are quite different from yours. You can be tagged as having one set of beliefs even though yours are almost the opposite.[4]

As the first COVID-19 contact-tracing apps were being introduced, Carmela Troncoso, a faculty member specializing in security and privacy at the Swiss École Polytechnique Féderalé de Lausanne, grew increasingly concerned. "I was not in favor of these apps because of the huge cost of surveillance," she said. "Privacy is not a goal in itself; it's a means to protect ourselves from what others learn about us." Nor were the apps themselves the only thing on Troncoso's mind. With infections soaring, some governments were considering issuing "immunity passports," documents attesting that someone had already had the disease and was therefore presumably immune (this turned out not to be the case). Looking at the range of information being collected on databases related to tracing and treating COVID-19, Troncoso stated, "That infrastructure should not be built."[5]

Yet Troncoso and other privacy researchers believed privacy-protective technology could play a role in containing the global pandemic. Could an app go backwards in time and check a person's proximity history while keeping the history of encounters private? Could the app send notifications to close contacts while keeping confidential who had exposed them to the disease? A number of cryptographers and privacy researchers around the world, Troncoso among them, saw a way to do this.

Three groups of researchers, one in Europe and two largely based in the United States, independently began developing a model based on essentially the same technical solution. Meanwhile, Google and Apple, who between them control the operating systems for almost all the world's smartphones, were thinking along similar lines. Collectively, all these groups were exploring the idea of apps that could provide information on exposure without revealing any information on people's encounters. The app would be able to tell Aliyah that she's been exposed to COVID-19 and was at risk of contracting the disease, but it would give no information that Bobby had exposed her to COVID-19—or even that they had been in each other's presence.[6]

This approach presented some engineering challenges common to all contact-tracing apps as well as some new ones. All of the solutions relied on BLE technology, but Apple's operating systems use proprietary technology for BLE signals running within their own apps. This saves battery life, but also prevents iPhone apps from communicating with Android devices if the apps were running in background.

The engineers needed to devise a system that would allow a privacy-protective proximity checking app to scan for signals every few minutes across operating systems without draining the battery. One option, of using a system-compatible app to wake up the phone's central processing unit to initiate scanning, would also drain the battery. The easy fix was to have the phone's operating system, which already manages this functionality for other applications, also do so for proximity-checking apps. This preserves the battery while ensuring that phones running different operating systems could conduct proximity checks.[7]

This solution provided an added benefit: Google and Apple could limit access to the infrastructure supporting this surveillance capability to "appropriate" apps. The companies agreed that only apps developed by public health agencies for the sole purpose of informing users of COVID-19 exposure could use the interoperable, proximity-checking, battery-preserving system; these apps would not be allowed to collect location information and would not be permitted to link from this app to other data without the user's explicit consent.[8]

Privacy was foremost in the cryptographers' minds. They focused on developing apps that reported exposures but not encounters—a different aim than that of either TraceTogether or Aarogya Setu. Instead of letting public health authorities know that Bobby had been infectious when he and Aliyah had encountered each other, the app would directly notify Aliyah she'd been exposed. That's all Aliyah would learn. She wouldn't know who or when, or even learn the list of encounters. Nor would anyone else.

The app might advise Aliyah to call her health department or doctor. It might recommend that she isolate herself and check her symptoms daily. The app might suggest testing. But unless Aliyah opted in to alert public health authorities to her potential exposure, public health authorities would not learn of Aliyah's exposure—and most people follow the default settings.

Technically, this was not a contact-tracing system; what Google, Apple, and the cryptographers had created was a system for exposure notification. The name the effort adopted, Google Apple Exposure Notification (GAEN), clarified that. A GAEN-based app would inform Aliyah, and only Aliyah, of her exposure.

In this model, privacy wins. No one learns of Bobby and Aliyah's encounter. Confidentiality wins too; Aliyah does not learn that Bobby exposed her to COVID-19. Public health authorities lose out, for such an app would not provide information to track the path of an epidemic. Without knowing how or where an infection is spreading, public health authorities have limited tools at their disposal for containing an epidemic. Public health authorities are not thrilled about this development.[9]

Epidemiologists use information from contact tracers to track how a disease is spreading and to determine where to put resources. "Suppose you are notified of a case in an apartment complex," Dr. Richard Rothenberg, Regents Professor at the Georgia State School of Public Health, told me. "You can test within the complex [for spread is likely there]." GAEN-based apps inform a person of exposure, but they don't tell them where or when the exposure took place. Even if Aliyah chooses to inform public health authorities that she's been exposed, she can't share information about where she became infected with them—*because she herself doesn't know.* Epidemiologists learn nothing about where spread is occurring.[10]

Keeping contact tracers out of the loop also has costs. "Sometimes people think contact tracing is about simply giving someone a phone call and giving them advice and expecting them to follow it," said Kate Adern, Director of Public Health in Wigan, England. She explained, "Whereas those of us who've got some experience in contact tracing know that the phone call is just the start. You've actually got to help that individual manage the consequences of the advice you're giving—if you want people to actually comply with the advice. That has been missed in the national thinking, not recognizing that, for example, if people work in the gig economy or they're self-employed, it's much more difficult to be off work for fourteen days." With an exposure notification system, public health departments could provide Aliyah support—but only if she reaches out to them and only if the local/state system has support to offer, which may not be the case. If Aliyah chooses not to, she's on her own.[11]

Why did the cryptographers and companies settle on exposure notification rather than a more traditional contact-tracing model? Privacy. If Ben is using TraceTogether when he is discovered to have COVID-19, his close contacts are shared with Singapore's Ministry of Health. If Aliyah is using a GAEN-based app, she learns of her exposure—but no one else does. No third party makes use of the fact that Aliyah and Bobby have been in close proximity. No one learns who Aliyah or Bobby's close contacts are. That's the way the cryptographers and the two tech companies wanted it.

Let's take a closer look at one of the GAEN-based apps. The European effort, DP3T, grew out of conversations between epidemiologists and cryptographers in Germany and Switzerland. SwissCovid, a Swiss GAEN-based exposure-notification app, was launched in June 2020.

As with all GAEN-based apps, SwissCovid relies on temporary identifiers to register users' proximity. These change frequently (every fifteen minutes), as do TraceTogether's but not Aarogya Setu's. A key difference between the GAEN system and TraceTogether, however, is that GAEN decentralizes all information public health authorities learn about people's exposures. As with all GAEN-based systems, the phones themselves generate the identifiers; unless at some point a phone shares its identifiers, only the phone that generated the identifier has information on which phone—and thus which person—the identifier belongs.

Suppose Amelie and Bart are both using the app and encounter each other when, unbeknownst to Bart, he is already infectious with COVID-19. Bart's identifier is stored on Amelie's phone for ten days, the incubation period for COVID-19.

Sometime after his encounter with Amelie, Bart feels ill and is tested for COVID-19. When Bart tests positive, he receives a verification code from the health authority to enter into the app. His phone uses this code to confirm with the health authority server that Bart has tested positive. Bart's phone then uploads the identifiers his phone used during his infectious period to the health department server.[12]

You might wonder why Bart's identifiers are uploaded to the server; after all, the health department already knows Bart is ill. The server needs Bart's identifiers to let those who came into contact with him know that they have potentially been infected—and it needs to do this without informing anyone that Bart may be the one who exposed them.

Amelie's SwissCovid app automatically checks with the health authority server twice daily to discover whether she has been exposed to COVID-19. If Amelie's time near Bart was short—say, less than ten minutes—she is not notified of possible exposure (based on current epidemiological knowledge, ten minutes is not long enough for her to become infected). But if Amelie encountered Bart for longer than that and was within six feet of him during that time, the app would alert her. As is the case for all GAEN-based apps, SwissCovid will not tell Amelie who exposed her, or even where she was exposed, but it will let her know that she needs to take precautions.

SwissCovid—and many other apps—can handle more complex situations as well. With COVID-19, your total exposure to the virus in a given period matters much more than who exposed you to the disease. Three five-minute exposures from different people in a short time period carries the same risk as a single, fifteen-minute exposure by one person with the same viral load. While the SwissCovid app cannot of course know a given person's viral load or what exactly you were doing when you were exposed, it attempts to solve for this problem by calculating a user's *total* exposure within a given twenty-four-hour period.

Let's say, for example, that the day Amelie encountered Bart was the same day that she also stood close to Chiara, Daniel, and Ella on the bus. All three were using SwissCovid, so Amelie's phone received their temporary identifiers as well. Amelie was on the bus for fifteen minutes, and she came into proximity with Chiara, Daniel, and Ella for less than ten minutes each. There's some variability in that measurement; Androids sample every three and a half to four minutes and iPhones every five.[13]

Two of Amelie's encounters that day—the ones with Daniel and Ella—turn out to be significant. A day after Bart tested positive, Daniel and Ella did as well. When Daniel and Ella entered their verification codes, their apps uploaded their temporary identifiers to the health authority's server. At that point the health authority's server has the temporary identifiers for Bart, Daniel, and Ella during the period each was infectious.[14]

Each check-in by the SwissCovid app actually asks ten questions of the server. Which identifiers were uploaded ten days ago? Which were uploaded nine days ago? Which eight days ago? And so on, up to the previous twenty-four hours. Amelie's app then calculates whether Amelie had a cumulative exposure of fifteen minutes within any of the twenty-four-hour periods. If yes, Amelie receives an alert from the app that tells her to call the Infoline and avoid contact with other people for ten days. She's also told she's eligible for free COVID-19 testing.[15]

What happens next is up to Amelie. There's no legal requirement for Amelie to call Infoline or isolate. Even if there were, it would be unenforceable, since the health authorities are not informed of Amelie's exposure. But Amelie has an incentive to call. The Swiss government makes isolation easier by providing financial support if Amelie has received an alert through the app, but Amelie has to reach out for this to happen. Because exposure notification doesn't let anyone but Amelie know of her risk, Amelie misses out on a contract tracer's encouragement and potential support unless she herself initiates it. How Amelie responds to the exposure notification is entirely her choice.[16]

SwissCovid was the first GAEN-based app, but it's hardly the only one (and more are arriving all the time). Because the apps are developed by different public health authorities, their variations reflect local preferences—with the firm caveat that location is never collected.

The Republic of Ireland's COVID Tracker Ireland combines the privacy protections of an exposure-notification app with an option that provides some of the benefits of contact tracing. When users sign up, they are given a choice whether their potential exposures can be shared with public health authorities, thereby enabling some contact-tracing features.

Like Aarogya Setua, COVID Tracker Ireland also has a daily check-in function for users. The Irish version is far more specific than the Indian version. The survey starts by asking users to pick either "I'm good, no symptoms," or "I'm not feeling well today." If a user marks that she's not feeling well, she's asked about fever, coughing, trouble breathing, or loss of sense of taste or smell. The app provides some basic medical advice based on a user's entries and keeps a record of symptoms over the past twenty-eight days.[17]

If a COVID Tracker Ireland user, Aoife, has opted into the contact-tracing system, she will have provided a phone number at the time she signed up for the app. If Aoife receives an exposure notification, so does the health department, and Aoife will be called by a contact tracer. Otherwise, Aoife will simply receive an exposure notification, more or less like SwissCovid's. In either case, no one learns who caused her exposure.[18]

The app appears to be surprisingly popular: in its first week, 37 percent of Ireland's population downloaded the app. And in a sweet victory for public health and borderless worlds, Ireland's COVID Tracker interoperates with the exposure-notification app developed by Northern Ireland.[19]

COVID Tracker Ireland has another feature as well. With the user's permission, it collects various types of metrics, including whether the app is in use, whether the user has been notified of exposure, and the ratio of such alerts to positive tests. Ireland's Health Services and Department of Health use this information in the aggregate to determine the app's impact on curtailing the disease. If such information is not collected—and most GAEN-based apps don't do so—there's no way to measure the apps' effectiveness.[20]

Both Switzerland and Ireland developed a single GAEN-based app for the nation. In the United States, public health is almost entirely the responsibility of state and local governments— and that means the apps have been too. In the US this responsibility falls to the states, and the IT departments of state public health agencies have been responsible for developing—or contracting out the development of—contact-tracing apps. Various states are developing GAEN-based apps, with Virginia's first out of the gate in early August 2020.

The existence of potentially fifty different exposure-notification apps in a country with porous internal borders creates complexity. What happens if Bobby, who lives in Washington state and works in Oregon, uses a Washington GAEN-based app and encounters Aliyah in Portland, where she lives and uses an Oregon GAEN-based app? To find out if she's been exposed to the coronavirus, Aliyah's Oregon-based app needs to check not just the temporary identifiers reported to the Oregon state health authorities, but also those reported to Washington and to other states.

Although the state apps vary in how they work—think of the differences between SwissCovid and COVID Tracker Ireland— they retain the key features of all GAEN-based apps. The app itself calculates risk of exposure; temporary identifiers are generated by users' phones; and users' identities are uploaded to a central server only after a confirmed COVID-19 test. This means that all the Oregon app needs to know is which Washington temporary identifiers belong to someone who tested positive (and the Washington app needs to know the same thing about the Oregon temporary identifiers). If Bobby was tested while in San Francisco, the Washington app would have to accept the verification code issued by California's Department of Public Health. The national organization for state and local public health labs, the Association of Public Health Laboratories (APHL), is working on a cloud-based solution enabling state and territorial public health GAEN-based apps to interoperate.[21]

The European Union is creating an infrastructure that will effectively erase national borders for European apps that meet certain standards for privacy protection. To qualify, apps must be voluntary, decentralized, transparent, and secure; use temporary identifiers; and not collect location data. An app downloaded in one country will be able to report a positive COVID-19 test conducted in a second nation and receive exposure notifications while in a third. That's ease of use and privacy in a single package.[22]

Privacy was the driving force of the GAEN-based apps, but as Troncoso noted, privacy is simply a means for protecting ourselves from the consequences of what others might do with the information they learn about us. In acting to protect privacy, we need to understand three different issues: Who might want to know about me? What might they want to learn? And what might they do with the information?[23]

Let's start with the "who." The public has a great appetite for information for well-known people—even if they are well known only within a small community. People who know you are also potentially interested; this ranges from people at work to casual acquaintances to friends and family. And while many people say, "I have nothing to hide," the fact is that most of us use some type of curtains in our homes and do not publish our tax returns or love letters. We selectively choose what information we share with our spouses, our children, our parents, our friends, and in the workplace, and consider it healthy to do so.[24]

The exposure-notification apps reveal only that we may have been exposed to the disease; contact-tracing apps combine this information with intelligence on whom we spend our time with. If we're focused on health-related information, the pool of potentially interested parties increases dramatically, including employers—present and potential—and health authorities. If a jurisdiction enforces quarantine, law enforcement may also want to know. Meanwhile, epidemiologists are interested in the information for both public health and research.

What might these various parties want to do with this information? Friends and family are always curious about the choices people make in their daily lives: who they see, where they go, what they do. Governments regularly seek information about where we are and whom we meet. Sometimes it's for such purposes as planning (for instance, revising bus and subway schedules); sometimes it's for use in criminal and national security investigations. Some governments, including the US and the UK, also track the movements and associations of people involved in political and civil society groups. The explosion of online advertising means that the private sector, too, is now intensely interested in our whereabouts and our social networks.[25]

During a pandemic, governments want to know if people are obeying quarantine and social distancing rules. Public health and medical authorities want to learn how the disease progresses and the effectiveness of particular treatments. Epidemiologists want to track a disease's spread and where future hot spots might be brewing. And everyone wants to know which groups are most vulnerable to the disease. Answering those questions requires a lot of data, much of it highly personal.

As for what people do with the information they learn, that depends. Family members might become upset over their relatives' choices to go to a bar or large party. Or they might be relieved to know that a loved one was not exposed at work, even though there had been an infected person on the factory floor. Universities might use the information to warn a student of exposure. Or they might use the information to expel a student who failed to follow the rules about no large gatherings. Governments might decide to provide financial support to induce exposed people to stay home. They might decide to use the information to close certain locations that are too crowded.[26]

This information is quite powerful; that's why the GAEN-based apps limit sharing of information. But even though GAEN has built a system to protect privacy, any contact-tracing or exposure-notification app, including GAEN-based apps, requires that at least some users (those who test positive) upload temporary identifiers onto a publicly accessible server. How secure is the server? How secure is the process? Are there strong protections against a rogue employee releasing information? When a system says it anonymizes data before releasing it, does the anonymization process really work?

An initial step is for app developers and public health agencies to provide clear and explicit statements about the processes of how data is handled and where it is stored. Specificity matters; a privacy policy that says "we keep your data safe" can mean anything. Does the policy explicitly state where the data is stored, who has access to it, and under what circumstances? This enables organizations like India's Internet Freedom Foundation and the press to see whether the app's owners are actually adhering to the stated policy.[27]

We know, for instance—because it said so publicly—that APHL plans to store identifiers provided by individual state and territorial agencies on a Microsoft cloud. This explicit answer is useful. While some might worry about such highly personal data being stored in a commercial service, most experts consider the Microsoft cloud to be secure and privacy-protective. Even the US Department of Defense, known for its focus on security, relies on the Microsoft cloud for government computing.

Seeing is believing. It's not good enough to know how the app works; for data as private and personal as that collected by contact-tracing and exposure-notification apps, accountability depends on being able to check that the computer code does what the app provider claims. That's why the code should be "open source," that is, publicly visible. The two GAEN apps we've discussed, SwissCovid and COVID Tracker Ireland, are open source, as is TraceTogether, whose code then became the basis for Australia's COVIDSafe app. With open source, someone else can use the code to create an app, but the app can't use the GAEN infrastructure unless it is from a public health authority. But while Aarogya Setu's app code is public, its server code is not, thus limiting the public's ability to evaluate the developers' stated claims about security and privacy.[28]

You can't keep information private if you don't first secure it. The questions about security raise many of the same issues as the broad privacy questions do—Who might want to know about me? What might they want to learn? And what might they do with the information?—but the focus is from a somewhat different angle.

Security experts are not worried about a curious friend who wants to know whom you were with the previous evening (the friend's best bet is to look at the phone when you're out of the room). Security experts are concerned about an adversary who seeks to hurt you or your community. And the adversary may be willing to use illegal methods to get at the information. Your information may not even be the end goal; it might simply be a stepping-stone to someone else's. That means it's not always clear who your attacker might be.

Contact-tracing and exposure-notification apps are, in theory, enormously efficient tools to determine when someone may have been exposed to someone or some people who later tested positive for COVID-19. We would do well, however, to remember that any efficiency has a cost. In trying to combat COVID-19 through the use of technology, we've created a new security risk: new forms of personal data, some of it on phones, and richer sources in the databases.

What might the attackers want to learn? Adversaries can have very targeted goals, as in the case of the Chinese hackers who stole the personnel records of 21 million people from the US Office of Personnel Management. The scope of the theft included not only all federal employees but also anyone who had applied for a government security clearance. Records included financial data, psychological records, and information on drug and alcohol use, information that could open the targets to blackmail—and now it was in the hands of the Chinese government. Someone executing a targeted attack on contact-tracing or exposure-notification information might be looking for who's infected or who's spending time with whom, or they might be seeking to know where infection is spreading to corner the market on masks or other forms of protective equipment.

It's also possible that an adversary might simply be exploring what kinds of information they can stow away for later use. An attacker might simply want to know the identity of your evening companion—blackmail, anyone?—but they might not stop at that. Apps that centralize information offer attackers the opportunity to learn the temporary identifiers of anyone you've encountered, and possibly where you've been.

Adversaries can also come from inside national security or law enforcement. Some NSA employees used internal databases collected for terrorism investigations to check on the communications of lovers and exes. Contact-tracing and exposure-notification apps collect information on infection and encounters. Law-enforcement investigators might pressure a health authority into releasing information about encounters in a critical criminal investigation. Despite their public commitments to using collected data only for public health purposes, centralized systems such as TraceTogether or Aarogya Setu could be subject to this sort of interagency pressure. GAEN-based and privacy-protective proximity-checking systems are designed to ensure that information about encounters instead resides on individuals' phones.[29]

Some security experts also worry that contact-tracing and exposure-notification apps offer opportunities to sow disinformation. If large numbers of people falsely reported positive COVID-19 diagnoses, especially after being in crowded situations—an outdoor football game or political protest, for example—lots of people would receive false notices of exposure. Some would unnecessarily isolate themselves; some would discover the deceit. Trust in the apps, and in the health care system, would decrease. The apps' designers anticipated and eliminated that particular problem by requiring a verification code from the health authorities for a positive COVID-19 test before sending out notification. But like any security threat, attackers are likely to return with a different form of attack.[30]

One can envision multiple other attacks, some more plausible, some less so. Some will undoubtedly be deployed. The best of the contact-tracing and exposure-notification apps minimize insecurity, but they can't entirely eliminate the risk. Any time there is a data collection system, there will be attacks. Some may succeed.

Securing the system means protecting against all these types of issues, and more. It involves all the standard ways of protecting computer systems—ensuring that users are authenticated, encrypting communication and stored data, protecting against insiders leaking information—and some new ones. These new forms of data use present new risks.

Contact-tracing apps are premised on the idea that technology can help solve an intractable problem. The coronavirus's ability to be transmitted through the air, even by people not experiencing symptoms, posed frightening risks to public safety. The result was two simultaneous crises: the COVID-19 pandemic and the economic crisis spawned by "stay home, stay safe" orders. Stay-at-home orders helped lower the damage from the first, but they created and exacerbated the second. In this context, contact-tracing apps and their privacy-protective cousin, exposure-notification apps, promise to make it easier for people to make decisions about venturing out—including going to work.

In theory, a tool that can go back in time to recall interactions between people provides a way to lower the infection rate. If Aliyah followed the suggestion to isolate, her use of an app could potentially break some COVID-19 transmission chains. In practice, the situation is somewhat more complicated. There are complexities ranging from how well the apps work in varied environments—on a train, in an apartment building, in a lecture hall—and what impact they have on a disease with a high percentage of asymptomatic carriers. We now turn to the critical issue of efficacy.

5 CAN CONTACT-TRACING APPS BE EFFECTIVE TOOLS OF PUBLIC HEALTH?

To stop an epidemic, public health authorities focus on lowering R_0. Even for a given illness, this number varies tremendously according to the protective measures a society takes (wearing masks, practicing social distancing, and other measures). In early March 2020, COVID-19's R_0 was just below 4 in New York State. Once the state instituted a shelter-in-place order and virtually no one was on the streets, R_0 dropped below 1. It continued to hover quite close to 1 for the summer and into the fall, even after the state came back to life and began to open bars and restaurants.[1]

By helping to keep spread in check, could contact-tracing apps have lowered R_0 enough to allow people to safely work, participate in social life, and be with their families? Lacking a real-life human experiment to answer this question, epidemiologists turn to models; these are in turn based on existing data. In the case of COVID-19, some of the best data comes from a citizen-science app developed by the BBC to accompany its 2018 documentary on the Spanish flu, *Contagion! The BBC4 Pandemic*. Participants agreed to provide a twenty-four-hour snapshot of their locations and self-reported contacts, which epidemiologists then used to model how a similar epidemic would spread in twenty-first-century Britain.[2]

The BBC database ultimately included the locations and contacts of 36,000 people. It showed their movements over the course of a day, including how many people they saw at work, at school, and elsewhere. The data allowed researchers to develop a model that could simulate various interventions at the population level, from isolation, testing, contact tracing, and social distancing to app usage.[3]

The resulting model showed that if 90 percent of ill people self-isolated and their household quarantined upon learning of their infection, 35 percent of cases would have already spread the disease to another person. If 90 percent of the contacts of those infected also isolated upon learning of the previous person's infection, only 26 percent of cases would have infected someone else. The contact tracers, in other words, bought time. By having potentially infected people isolate, contact tracing prevented new rounds of infections. In another iteration, the researchers added apps to the mix and assumed that 53 percent of the population would use them. By notifying people of potential infections faster than a contact tracer could, the apps lowered the infection rate further, so that only 23 percent of cases infected another person. At that high adoption rate, the disease doesn't disappear, but it also doesn't cause a pandemic.[4]

Models, of course, are only as good as the assumptions on which they're based. The idea that 53 percent of any given population would voluntarily use a contact-tracing app and that anyone receiving an exposure notification would isolate is doubtful, at best. Still, because the apps appear to help lower R_0, governments and public health officials have jumped to add them to the mix of public health tools available to combat COVID-19's spread.[5]

Given the high stakes involved, we need to look at how apps are deployed in real life. How well do apps actually work? Are they more effective than more traditional, and less invasive, public health tools? Can they usefully supplement manual contact-tracing efforts? COVID-19 has hit low-income and Black, Latinx, and indigenous communities particularly hard. The possibility of public health organizations embracing contact-tracing apps as a line of defense against epidemics raises new questions about equity and the balance of individual privacy and public safety. Will contact-tracing apps exacerbate inequities already present in society?

A robust public debate about the implications of deploying what is effectively a public surveillance system didn't occur; instead, many officials deployed these apps essentially overnight. We need that debate, but first we must look at efficacy. If the apps aren't efficacious, then there is no reason to consider them further.[6]

Following advice from the WHO, most public health agencies have promoted the idea that "social distancing" is the safest way to guard against exposure to the coronavirus. For the CDC, the magic number is six feet (in metric-based nations, it's usually two meters). Stay at least that far away from other people, so the theory goes, and you're safe. Since the BLE technology on which contact-tracing apps run depends on proximity, engineers hoped that phone-to-phone contacts could serve as a reasonable proxy for risky exposures. In practice, this has turned out to be not entirely straightforward.[7]

In theory, the strength of the BLE signal that a phone receives from another indicates the distance of the device emitting it. To test the accuracy of this assumption, researchers at Germany's Fraunhofer-Gesellschaft simulated the experiences of people sitting on a train, waiting on line, being served by a waiter in a restaurant, and attending a cocktail party. Over 139 tests, the phones correctly determined time and distance exposure

70 percent of the time. This information seems encouraging, but the simulation took place in a test facility that lacked walls. The "train car" had no metal sides, the people waiting on line encountered no checkout counters or supermarket shelves, and neither the restaurant nor the cocktail party included walls or serving stations. This matters because radio waves often reflect off surfaces.[8]

When researchers from the University of Dublin tried these tests in actual train cars, they obtained different results. Seven volunteers with phones running GAEN-based apps distributed themselves around a train car and measured the signals their phones received over a fifteen-minute period. Radio waves are supposed to vary inversely according to the square of distance, so the researchers were surprised to find that the signals stayed constant at a distance of 1.5–2.5 meters and began to *increase* after that. Apparently, a flexible metal joint between train carriages concentrated the signal.[9]

As they looked more closely at the results, the researchers found more surprises. Signal strength varied depending on whether a person carried their phone in their back pocket, their front pocket, or in a backpack or handbag. The signal strength varied by device model, by the shape of the room, even by the construction materials. Depending on the construction material, BLE signals can indicate that people are near each other when they are actually in neighboring apartments.[10]

Epidemiologists understand that the six-foot measure is somewhat arbitrary; engineers know that BLE signals don't measure distances precisely. If the rest of us come to use these systems, we also need to understand their limitations.

Measurement imprecision isn't the only problem for contact-tracing and exposure-notification apps. The apps are not built to record the real-life circumstances that affect the likelihood of transmission in any given case. If Alyssa is six feet away from Ben in a small room for fifteen minutes, there's likely risk of exposure. But if Alyssa is four feet from Ben, outside, and wearing a mask, she's likely to be safe. Large gatherings of people indoors carry risks of spread, while similarly sized groups of masked people outdoors are less dangerous. Apps can't distinguish between these situations. Nor do apps know if the person standing eight feet away from you is belting out a song—dangerous if they're infected—or just standing quietly.

The apps are also ignorant of a room's ventilation, an important factor in how the virus spreads. When an infected person breathes—or speaks, sings, coughs, or sneezes—they emit viral particles packaged in a mixture of mucus, saliva, and water. The smallest of these, aerosols, evaporate as they travel, losing some of their potency. The bigger ones, droplets, typically fall to the ground within three feet. Sometimes, though, air flow, particularly air conditioning, can push these along, putting people at further distances at risk of infection. This is apparently what happened in a restaurant in Guangzhou, China, when two people sitting well beyond the six-foot measure—and on different sides of the ill person—were infected. One was at a table more than a dozen feet away.[11]

Biology also confuses apps. A review of published reports indicates that as many as 30–40 percent of people never show symptoms. While these studies are not based on random samples, a single study based on a large random sample of Icelanders showed a similar result: a startling 43 percent of participants tested positive without showing symptoms. Even if one assumes that only 30 percent of cases are asymptomatic—a not unreasonable assumption—then epidemiologists believe that 7 percent of transmission will arise from asymptomatic cases. This matters for the apps' effectiveness. Asymptomatic people are less likely to get tested than those who are sick—and if there's no test, there's no trigger for exposure notifications.[12]

Contact-tracing and exposure-notification apps nevertheless do have value. They pick up cases that people, including contact tracers, wouldn't. Aliyah might not remember a chance hallway encounter with Bobby, but her app will. And the app will be ready to notify Aliyah if Bobby's phone reports a positive COVID-19 test. Perhaps even more critically, Aliyah's app will register encounters with nearby strangers in the bar or theater lobby—as long as they are also using the app. If those strangers later test positive, Aliyah will learn she's been exposed. Without a phone app, she'd have little chance of discovering this.

These technical and practical limitations of contact-tracing apps mean that they can produce both false positives and false negatives. (Note that these are false positives and false negatives *of exposure*, not false positive and false negatives *of having COVID-19*.) Virginia's website for the state's GAEN-based app, for example, warns that students in adjacent dorm rooms might receive exposure notifications of close contact while being in different rooms. When tested in August 2020, the UK exposure-notification app had a 45 percent false positive rate and 31 percent false negative rate. These numbers sound bad, but the false positives aren't entirely "false"—most of them represented exposures at 2.5–4 meters away rather than 2 meters. Depending on the circumstances, a person might well have been exposed at 3 meters. In the case of false negatives, however, users received no notification whatsoever that they had been in the presence of someone infected with COVID-19.[13]

Both types of inaccuracies present challenges for users and public health agencies—some more obvious than others. If

Aliyah receives a false positive notification, she might quarantine unnecessarily, losing a paycheck. If she's following the rules, she should also urge her roommates and family members she's in close contact with to do so, causing more disruption. Alternatively, if this is the second time that the app warns Aliyah that she's been exposed without her developing any symptoms, she might just ignore the notification and disable the app.

False negatives place the public's health at risk. If Bobby was asymptomatic and never tested, Aliyah will not receive a notification even though she may have spent fifty minutes sitting six feet away from Bobby in a classroom. False negatives can also be produced by circumstance: from an air conditioner dispersing aerosols farther than expected or an infected singer who propels droplets farther than six feet.

Some communities are at higher risk for false positives than others. Many low-income people, for instance, hold jobs that bring them in constant contact with a stream of strangers (e.g., grocery store clerks, health care workers, workers in food service and production). For these workers, a small variation in the proximity measurement (say, nine feet instead of six) can multiply into a high risk of false positives from contact-tracing apps. What's more, many of these workers routinely wear protective gear or work behind barriers that reduce their risk from even four-foot interactions. Similarly, people who live in high-density housing situations, whether multifamily housing units or apartment complexes, are more likely to receive false positives than people who live in stand-alone suburban or rural houses.[14]

Hourly workers living paycheck to paycheck can't afford to take time off unless it's absolutely necessary. A false positive keeps them from clocking in. Alyssa, in Singapore, or Amelie, in Switzerland, can each expect to receive financial support from the government if they isolate after an exposure notification. But in the United States, few low-income or gig workers receive paid time off, even for isolating during a pandemic. The privilege of staying at home is not evenly distributed. Workers who realize that the apps consistently generate false positives are less likely to use them voluntarily—or to heed them when they provide alerts.

False negatives, too, have a differential impact. White-collar workers who already work from home and who drive their own vehicles on necessary errands have fewer contacts than those who take public transportation to jobs that have been deemed "essential." The fewer contacts each of us has with other people, the less chance we have of spreading COVID-19. A false negative of exposure for someone who works outside the home and uses public transit carries greater risk of infecting others than the same false negative for someone who works at home and uses their own transportation.

Contact-tracing apps were supposed to resolve this problem, allowing people to emerge from lockdowns with the ability to interact with friends, family, and strangers. But at least in the United States, the realities of socioeconomic inequality and racism are likely to limit the apps' effectiveness. To understand why, we need to take a closer look at how COVID-19 has spread through hard-hit communities.

Chelsea is a working-class city just across the Mystic River from Boston. The city has had an extremely high COVID-19 infection rate, five times higher than the state average and over three times higher than Boston's. One in five of Chelsea's residents lives below the federal poverty line. The area's dense housing and persistent poverty only partially explain Chelsea's high rate of COVID-19 infections. Much of this can only be explained by the effects of systemic racism.[15]

Chelsea's population is two-thirds Latinx, the demographic with the highest rate of infection in the United States. Many residents live in multigenerational households and a high percentage work in food services, many of which were deemed essential and stayed open during the pandemic. Almost half are recent immigrants. Looking at COVID infections across towns and cities in Massachusetts, researchers at Harvard T. H. Chan School of Public Health and Beth Israel Deaconess Medical Center found a strong correlation between these factors and high rates of COVID-19 infections.[16]

For immigrants, COVID-19 presents an additional set of challenges beyond the nearly universal worries about health and lost wages. In February 2020, the Trump administration enacted a rule denying green cards, visas, and citizenship to anyone who had used public aid. Though the so-called public charge rule has been waived during the COVID-19 crisis, noncitizens and those with noncitizen relatives feared its reinstatement at any time. One consequence is that many immigrants have avoided seeking public health care, a choice that inevitably leads to the disease's spread. People at risk make decisions they view as best for themselves and their families. In the case of COVID-19, those decisions may be right for the person but less than ideal for public health.[17]

The possibility of raids by Immigration and Customs Enforcement and the threat of deportation govern people's decisions, even during a pandemic. In Chelsea, few residents accepted the city's offer to use unoccupied hotel rooms as isolation quarters. "I think there is some uncertainty and anxiety that is inhibiting the flow of guests to the hotel, because it is attributed to the government," Alexander Train, assistant director of Chelsea's Department of Planning and Development, said. "It's about, 'what if I don't make it back to my family?'" With such fears ever present, immigrants are unlikely to use an app that tracks either their location or their contacts.[18]

COVID has also had a devastating effect on Black people living in the United States. Twenty-three percent of Chicago residents are Black, but in April, 58 percent of the city's COVID deaths were of Black people. By then, it had become clear that Black people in the United States were disproportionately dying from COVID. The causes were decades in the making, a result of structural racism.[19]

Due to generations of housing segregation, redlining practices, and public divestments, neighborhoods with majority Black residents have less healthy living conditions when compared with similarly situated white neighborhoods. Black Americans are more likely to reside in areas with multiunit residential buildings and more likely to use public transport, both factors putting them at greater risk of exposure. Decades of federal housing policies prevented Black families from moving into white neighborhoods. Discriminatory housing policies have resulted in Black neighborhoods being more heavily polluted, with Black Americans living in closer proximity to polluting facilities. Such unhealthy environments, especially those with high air pollution, creates a literally deadly risk when combined with COVID-19, a disease that attacks the respiratory system. Adding to this burden is the fact that many Black neighborhoods are also "food deserts." Instead of purchasing food at supermarkets purveying fresh fruit and vegetables, residents have to rely on convenience stores selling processed food—high in calories and low in nutrition.[20]

These structural factors contribute to Black Americans' high rates of chronic illness, including cardiovascular disease, diabetes, and hypertension, all of which correlate with poorer outcomes when people are infected with COVID-19. What's more, decades of tough-on-crime policies have disproportionately incarcerated Black Americans in jails and prisons, where overcrowding and limited hygiene and medical care contributes to the virus's spread. The result is that, at the time of this writing, nearly one in 1,000 Black Americans have been killed by the disease; the rate for white Americans is half that.[21]

Centuries of racism in the government and the medical profession have contributed to poor health outcomes for Black Americans; this mistreatment has, naturally enough, created layers of distrust of government and medical experts by the Black community. The Tuskegee study is only one of many examples in this history. Others include denying Black patients medical care and using Black bodies for medical research without permission. A 2002 Institute of Medicine study concluded that, for almost every disease, Black Americans received less effective treatment than did white Americans. Black Americans were less likely to receive routine medical procedures, were treated later in the course of disease (when a good prognosis is less likely), and were less likely to receive medical interventions. Such disparities in treatment lead to poorer outcomes. That's true even now for cases of COVID-19. Distrust of public health advice—and of disembodied apps—is a natural response in such situations.[22]

Contact tracing, whether conducted by public health workers or apps, doesn't work without trust. Successful contact tracers know this; they accompany their contact tracing with public health work. Howard Brown Health is a Chicago health care organization focusing on the LGBTQ population; 92 percent of its low-income Black and Latinx clients eventually tested positive for COVID-19. Contact tracers began their conversations with clients by asking, "How can we help you? What can we do right now to help you get by?" They provided infected patients with food deliveries—and sometimes cash—and assisted with housing so that infected people could socially distance.[23]

Convincing patients to participate in contact tracing also involves assuring them that the tracers will protect the confidentiality of information that patients share. Confidentiality is drilled into contact tracers' training. Johns Hopkins University's COVID-19 Contact Tracing course, for example, says that even if a contact tracer learns from a patient interview that her own family member's acquaintances may have been exposed to the disease, the tracer can't share the information with her relative—for doing so would violate confidentiality. (Of course, the contact tracer can remind her family members to practice safe social distancing.)[24]

Yet even while contact tracers are trained to emphasize that their work is driven by public health rather than public surveillance, many people, and particularly members of marginalized communities, prefer to minimize their contacts with government representatives. Some members of these communities perceive calls from contact tracers as a sign that "I'm being traced, I'm being tracked," said Tony Gillespie, vice president of public policy and engagement for the Indiana Minority Health Coalition. "Especially in racial and ethnic minority communities and Hispanic and Latino communities, that's a real concern."[25]

The current generation of contact-tracing apps was not built to address the specific needs of marginalized communities. The apps appear predicated on the model of a middle- or upper-class income and a job that can be done from home. They haven't been designed to accommodate the fears and skepticism of communities that has been oversurveilled and are often unable to take advantage of recommendations to stay home.

Zinzi Bailey, a social epidemiologist at the University of Miami Miller School of Medicine, told me, "A notice from an app, 'Oh, you may have been exposed' might not be so much of an issue for a Black middle-class person in an integrated neighborhood." Such a person could afford to stay home—and in fact may already have been working from home. The consequences for a person of color living in a segregated, impoverished community are quite different. "In a neighborhood of over policing [and lack of police when needed]," Bailey said, "and a higher percentage of people incarcerated—no." They won't use the app. Bailey explained, "An app is less likely to be used in marginalized communities because of lack of trust." Whether or not members of these communities are willing to use an app will also depend in large part on whether law enforcement or immigration authorities either will have or are perceived to have access to the information.[26]

Contact tracing is merely a means to lowering R_0 and the disease's spread. To ask whether an app does this successfully is not to ask whether the app can uncover cases people can't—it can. The question is whether the app can lower R_0. That depends on how many people use the app and whether people actually follow an app's notifications to isolate. As we have seen, the reasons a person might choose either to not use or to ignore an app are plentiful and powerful. This takes us right back to where we started: human contact tracing.

Human-based contact tracing brings community insight and care in a way impossible to package in a phone. We see this clearly in the case of the Fort Apache Indian Reservation in eastern Arizona. The reservation is home to the White Mountain Apache Tribe, who are strongly connected to the land and are guardians of its ponderosa pine forests and the remains of the Kinishba pueblo, a remarkable archeological site dating from the mid-twelfth to the mid-fourteenth century. The reservation also has persistently high poverty levels, and many of its residents live with chronic disease. Given this, you'd expect to see high infection and mortality rates for COVID-19. And in fact many people were infected—but few died. Despite a chronic lack of funding, the medical team at the Whiteriver Indian Hospital (part of the Indian Health Service) were able to mount an early-response plan that saved lives. It relied heavily on in-person contact tracing.[27]

At Fort Apache, families tend to live in multigenerational homes. In contrast to Anglo families, grandparents, especially grandmothers, have significant responsibility for raising the grandchildren. Children in Apache families may stay with their nonresident grandmother for extended periods. Instead of asking infected patients, "Where have you been?," contact tracers queried, "Who are your grandparents?" If someone was infected with the coronavirus, contact tracers checked out the health of both sets of grandparents—even if one set didn't share the household.[28]

While the large distances on the reservation might, in theory, limit the spread of the disease through the community at large, the family structure raises the risk of clusters and creates challenges for treatment. With individual homes frequently crowded, a single sick family member can lead to multiple illnesses. Meanwhile, with hospitals as much as an hour's drive away, those who are infected may not be able to get to help when they need it. COVID-19 tends to be a mild illness unless and until it's not. One symptom, known as "happy hypoxia," is particularly dangerous: a person might feel fine, even as their blood-oxygen saturation level plummets to 60 or even 50 percent. Then, suddenly, they're gasping for breath. With COVID, early intervention can be the difference between life and death.[29]

Because contact tracers knew all this, they checked the oxygen saturation levels for everyone living in a household with an ill person. By doing this, they found people with saturation levels of 80 percent who had been unaware that they had any sort of health problem. Notice how different this is from traditional contact tracing: instead of starting with a person who tested positive for the coronavirus, and then encouraging that person's contacts to get tested, too, the contact tracers skipped the test and went straight to the symptoms. When the disease was peaking, one in five households had someone who would be hospitalized because of low oxygen levels.[30]

These interventions, in other words, were less about contact tracing and more about saving lives—which is, of course, the ultimate goal of contact tracing. It appears to have worked. Despite the reservation's high infection rate, its death rate was lower than the state's. This intervention was grueling and staff-intensive; it worked because the contact tracers understood their community's social structure. The medical teams included community volunteers who knew "the language, the people, [and] the community." Contact tracers working with the Fort Apache Reservation ask questions that save grandparents' lives.[31]

What would it take for apps to work as well as the Fort Apache contact tracers? Obviously, all three legs of the contact-tracing tripod—test, trace, and isolate—have to be working, but the requirements are deeper than that. The entire public health apparatus has to be working properly, which means that facilities are available when people need them. Trust is essential; without that, people won't share information with human contact tracers.

Compared with having a public health system that works for everyone, creating an effective public health apparatus to test, trace, and isolate seems like the easy part. However, six months into the pandemic, this has not yet happened. A surprising number of wealthy, supposedly technically advanced countries have failed to master the art of readily available, low-cost COVID-19 testing. In Germany, testing has been easy to obtain, with results typically back in thirty-six hours. France has been less consistent—results could take that time, or take up to a week. In the UK, as students returned to school and people to work, the testing system was overwhelmed, with only 14 percent of tests returned within twenty-four hours. Backlogs are anticipated to continue at least through the winter of 2020–2021, a year after the pandemic began. In October 2020, the US was still performing only 70 percent of the testing considered necessary to stop the spread of the disease, and backlogs continued.[32]

Singapore and Korea tackled the "trace" part of the triad, successfully tracking down contacts by phone. That model has proved less successful in the West. The *Wall Street Journal* reported that people who tested positive often failed to respond to contact tracers' calls. Annoyed about spam calls, many people don't answer their phones unless they recognize the number. New York State was doing well, reaching 90 percent of people who tested positive; New Jersey was reaching 70 percent; Connecticut, 90 percent. In other locations, however, the numbers have been less good. In Maryland and Louisiana, contact tracers have reached fewer than two out of every three people who have tested positive; in Los Angeles County, closer to half.[33]

Those Americans who did answer a contact tracer's call often wouldn't reveal their contacts, sometimes even hanging up on contact tracers. Nor is this a uniquely American problem. In Taiwan, an infected person provides an average of fifteen names; in Spain, it is three. A third of contacted Philadelphians claimed they hadn't been in close contact with anyone, a response that defies belief. In one case involving an outbreak sparked by a party, New York State issued subpoenas before some of the partygoers "remembered" who else had been present.[34]

Isolation was also failing. Researchers in the UK discovered that only 18 percent of those who had COVID-like symptoms between March and August had isolated. The respondents said that they did not isolate because they needed to go out for food or medications—or just because they felt better. Men, young people, and those who needed to work because of low income or being in a key sector were those least likely to isolate. Lack of social services explains much of the rest. Who'll buy food if I isolate? Who'll pay my rent? Where can I stay so I don't infect my family? Who will take care of my kids or check on my parents? Without social provisions for making sure that people have access to food, rent, and a place to stay, it's no wonder that so few people isolate.[35]

Distrust of the government—or of government-provided health care—is part of the reason for the failures of test, trace, and isolate. The political polarization of the late 2010s, however, has created additional layers of mistrust that public health authorities worldwide have struggled to overcome. That's been extraordinarily difficult when compounded by multiple government failures, ranging from early lack of proper medical equipment to a continuing lack of testing facilities.

Let's presume, for a moment, that public health agencies and their partners in government implemented an effective infrastructure for test, trace, and isolate and convinced the public to participate. How would contact-tracing apps work within this system? As we've seen, apps are not a magic bullet: they produce both false positives and false negatives. A much bigger issue is the legitimate concerns that marginalized groups have over how government agencies might use their data. No number of privacy statements will resolve the distrust of government that many members of these communities have.

An app that fails to work for a given community is an app that fails us all. Indeed, the most effective public health tool is the one that is attuned to the communities most in need. The GAEN-based apps, which have been widely adopted in Europe and are being rapidly adopted in the United States, are not focused on such communities. GAEN-based apps only work on relatively new smartphones: Android 6.0+ (Marshmallow) or iOS 13.5 or above. Those who are most at risk—service workers, who are exposed to lots of people daily, and the elderly, who suffer the most serious consequences of a COVID-19 infection—are least likely to have phones that support the exposure-notification apps.[36]

An equitable app would be one that's accessible to low-income, minority, and elderly populations and built to accommodate the reality of their lives. As we've seen, these realities vary. Chelsea's Latinx population lives in multigenerational households and tight quarters; the White Mountain Apache live in multigenerational households whose members may shift by the week as children move between households. Black Chicagoans rely heavily on public transportation, while Native Americans living on reservations may need to drive several hours in a private vehicle to reach the nearest hospital. Each factor changes what risks a person faces, whether they would voluntarily use the app, and how a contact tracer should respond.

How, then, would we go about assessing apps' efficacy? We would have to begin by testing apps' efficacy in different communities, with different needs. The UK did that, testing the government's GAEN-based app, NHS Covid-19, on the Isle of Wight and in the London borough of Newham. In 2011, the last year for which official government figures are available, the non-white population of the Isle of Wight was 3 percent, a contrast from the UK's overall non-white population of 14 percent. In Newham, by contrast, 83 percent of the residents identify as Black, Asian, or minority ethnic. Residents of the Isle of Wight downloaded the app at three times the rate as did those in Newham. Was that because the Isle of Wight had been the subject of an earlier trial for the app, while it was completely new to the residents of Newham? Or do the differential download rates tell us something about racialized communities' willingness to share their personal information with a government agency?[37]

Another complicating factor involves how people's behaviors change over time. Efficacy is not something that can simply be tested once; rather, it must be continually assessed over the entirety of the app's use.

The very design of GAEN-based apps conspires against collecting the kinds of information that epidemiologists would need to evaluate their efficacy as a public health tool. Public health authorities know how many people have tested positive; they can compare the number of positive tests with the number of users who have uploaded identifiers to the public health server. This, at least, can tell them what percentage of the known-positive population is willing to participate in app-based exposure notification. But that's almost all they can learn about user behavior.

Researchers in Switzerland attempted to learn just this. When they looked at seven weeks' worth of SwissCovid data, they learned that 67 percent of the SwissCovid users who had tested positive had uploaded their temporary identifiers to public health servers. From that point, however, the trail went cold. They couldn't learn how many exposure notifications each positive report triggered, nor could they learn how many people quarantined after receiving an exposure notification. They could learn how many people went for tests after an exposure notification, but not the ratio of alerts to actual new cases (and thus how useful the apps actually are).[38]

The question is not whether the apps can notify someone about an exposure, encourage them to isolate, and stop a transmission route; there's no doubt that, in some instances, they will.

It's whether the apps are providing help to the communities most in need. And that's much harder to measure.

The privacy-protective cloak of GAEN-based exposure-notification apps fails to provide information about location, limiting the apps' value. This becomes especially important when dealing with the possibility of a so-called superspreading event. Earlier coronaviruses, like SARS, which caused an epidemic in 2002–2004, and MERS, which first appeared in 2012, largely spread via superspreaders. The pattern for COVID-19 appears to be similar.[39]

Many infected people don't spread the disease at all; 10 percent of cases appear to cause 80 percent of transmissions. Superspreading is most likely indoors, where there are lots of people, poor ventilation, and everyone sticks around for a relatively long period of time. Think of a cocktail party or a long movie, not a quick trip to the supermarket.[40]

To stop the pandemic's spread, we need to know much more than the likelihood that someone's been exposed. Shefali Oza, Data and Testing Manager at Partners in Health, explained, "Contact tracers want to find out context . . . if these contacts become a case [i.e., become infected], epidemiologists use that to find superspreaders." Did exposure happen within the close quarters of home, where spread is likely limited to family members? Or was the exposure from a superspreader? Exposure notification apps don't particularly help in answering this question.[41]

As an example, consider the cluster of COVID-19 cases associated with an outbreak at the White House. On October 1, White House senior counselor Hope Hicks, President Trump, and First Lady Melania Trump all tested positive for COVID-19. A day later, five more members of the president's inner circle tested positive. As the *Washington Post* noted, it's unlikely—though possible—that there were different sources of infection for those testing positive. The most likely explanation is that there was a superspreader present at some point during the September 26 Rose Garden announcement and subsequent indoor reception for US Supreme Court nominee Amy Coney Barrett. In this case, we have lots of information about who might have been exposed, as the event was widely covered by the media. We didn't need an app to tell us that several US senators and cabinet-level secretaries were likely exposed.[42]

Now imagine a scenario in which a contact-tracer is trying to understand a potential superspreader event in a less newsworthy situation, perhaps a conference taking place in a hotel. Imagine, as well, that the suspected superspreader is using a GAEN-based app. Close contacts using the app would learn of their exposure, though they wouldn't learn where or when they were exposed. Public health authorities would see an increase in positive tests. But until contact tracers actually interview infected contacts, no one would be able to put together that this was a superspreading incident. By then, the next round of exposures and infections would be well on their way. Privacy protections—the lack of location information—means that GAEN-based apps don't provide useful information for uncovering a superspreading incident.

Smartphones, those radios in our pocket, have changed the way we live and work. Today some of us expect to be able to get from here to there without first mapping the route or checking a bus schedule; others of us use the apps on our phones, instead of a field guide, to identify a scarlet tanager or purple love grass. The phones have become such an integral part of our daily lives that we have instituted social—and legal—norms to prevent their inappropriate use while sharing a meal or driving a car. Given phones' ubiquity, it was perhaps inevitable that technologists would see the devices as a natural solution to figure out who you might have infected during a pandemic. Some sought to do so in a way that protected privacy; the system that resulted has been embraced by a number of public health agencies around the world.

In designing the GAEN-based systems, Google and Apple effectively circumvented the public health system. Though the two companies have said that GAEN-based apps are intended to supplement contact tracing, the systems are not intended to work with contact tracers. Rather, as discussed in the previous chapter, they are tools for directly informing individuals of exposure.[43]

If aiding public health is the ultimate goal, why design in a way that bypasses contact tracing, a century-old system that is key to ending epidemics? The GAEN-based systems are not the only way that smartphone apps can help combat the spread of COVID-19. One alternative approach is to build apps that directly aid contact tracers in their work. Some, such as TraceTogether, do this, but their use of location information and personal contacts raises privacy concerns. But there are ways that new technology can aid contact tracers without introducing privacy risks. Because smartphones offer ubiquity, Internet connectivity, and mobility, they offer many features that could be useful to contact tracers that don't introduce such risks.

One tool takes advantage of a smartphone's role as a location tracker but gives users the option to control what information is shared. Common Circle, one of the US-based efforts in designing privacy-protective apps, developed an app, Assist, that jogs a user's memory by simplifying accessing meetings and location information that's available on a user's phone. Instead of making a user retrace their steps via Google Maps or asking them to review their calendar, the application assembles this data for the user. The data is shared *only with the user*, who then chooses what information to share with a contact tracer. There's no BLE technology, no proximity checking, and no new form of data collection. The app can't say who sat next to you on a bus, but it can remind you that you did, in fact, take the bus from 42nd and Fifth to 80th and Broadway last Tuesday and met Camila and Diego for coffee on Wednesday morning. It's a low-tech approach, easy to implement, and not privacy-invasive.[44]

Another tool helps alert a user when they've been in a hot spot. The UK's NHS COVID-19 app has a feature in which businesses, churches, and other venues display a QR code that users can scan when they visit. If Amelia goes to a pub, she can scan the NHS-supplied QR code, which is then stored in a diary on her phone. The code never leaves her phone. If the pub later discovers it was an infection hotspot, its QR code is uploaded to an NHS server. From that point, everything works much like proximity checking. Amelia's phone checks in with the NHS QR server several times a day, downloading identifiers of new hotspots. If there's a match with one stored on Amelia's phone, she discovers she's been in an infection hotspot and is advised to take appropriate steps.[45]

These approaches are not what engineers would call "sexy." They don't run on cool new technology or provide a fundamentally new way to combat disease. That might be a strength rather than a weakness. Apps of this sort don't raise new risks that centralized apps or location tracking apps do. They are widely deployable. And because the information stays entirely under a user's control, it doesn't raise privacy concerns. Others might— arguing for a set of guiding principles for the technology used for containing a disease.

The development of contact-tracing and exposure-notification apps opened the door to using technology that reveals highly personal aspects of our lives. Their deployment during the COVID-19 pandemic occurred in record speed. The public discussion of whether this is an appropriate public policy step did not. It's time to start it.

6 LOOKING TO THE LONG TERM

Public health authorities use the language of "surveil and contain" to describe their most powerful tool for ending an outbreak of infectious disease. Surveil to find the infected cases, then contain through isolation. This technique has been used for every known infectious disease for over a century. But in the early days of COVID-19, the words "surveil and contain" took on a more sinister cast. China used the full force of its surveillance network, which included drones, big data, and neighbors spying on neighbors (a tool from the days of Mao) to enforce a quarantine and contain the disease. By March, outbreaks of COVID-19 in China, Singapore, and South Korea appeared to be under control, even as infections and death rates soared in many locations on multiple continents.[1]

Western nations rejected the full force of China's surveillance network, but Singapore and South Korea demonstrated a willingness to enroll aspects of modern surveillance technologies in fighting disease. Singapore developed the TraceTogether system, and South Korea turned to cell tower records, CCTV, and credit card receipts. When Singapore released TraceTogether's source code, Australia adapted it for its own use (though the country later moved to a decentralized, GAEN-based system).

Germany, France, and the UK concurrently started efforts to develop their own centralized apps for contact tracing.

Privacy advocates began raising alarms about these apps while designs were still in the planning stage. In recent years, the European Union has strongly flexed its regulatory muscles to protect users' privacy. Centralized apps ran counter to these regulatory trends. Computer scientists, legal scholars, and epidemiologists on at least three continents began pressing for a privacy-protective, decentralized solution. In April 2020, the European Parliament opted for privacy, passing a resolution insisting that contact-tracing apps be decentralized. If public health authorities wanted to incorporate smartphone technology into their contact-tracing systems, they would have to do so in a privacy-protective way.[2]

Enter the Google–Apple partnership (GAEN). For these two companies, the decision to build infrastructure supporting proximity checking was a fraught one. While both companies were keen to provide technical assistance for ending the pandemic, they were also well aware that both states and private actors could use a proximity-checking infrastructure to spy on the most intimate aspects of individuals' lives. From the beginning, the companies instituted rules about how the apps could be used—only by public health authorities, and only under certain conditions. Apps would not be allowed to collect location information. They could not share users' identities with other apps. Users would control whether the app was activated—and could turn off the app at any time. The apps' infrastructure would be disabled in regions where the disease was no longer a threat.[3]

The GAEN system was developed rapidly. Google and Apple announced their effort in April 2020; the first GAEN-based app, SwissCovid, became available only two months later. Over the summer, other European public health authorities released their own exposure-notification apps. The first such app in the United States, Virginia's COVIDWISE, arrived in August 2020.[4]

For the first generation of exposure-notification apps, each public health agency developed its own, customized app using GAEN infrastructure. To speed up the process, in September 2020 Google and Apple created "Exposure Notification Express" (EN Express). This tool let public health agencies design an app through a menu of options provided by EN Express. "Public health wants to be expedient; it has a real lack of resources," Bill Darrow, a social epidemiologist with extensive experience at both the state level and the CDC, told me. "It can only fight one fire at a time." From a public health authority's perspective, any tool that would make it easier for them to focus on their agency's core functions would be a plus.[5]

With EN Express, states gained speed, but they lost control. Instead of using in-house expertise to customize their choices, state public health agencies were limited to the options offered by EN Express. Recall that COVID Tracker Ireland offered users the option of providing a phone number to allow contact tracers to reach out to those who had been exposed. EN Express didn't offer that option. A state may decide to include that option and could, instead, build its own GAEN-based app. But given the limited time and money that characterize most public health agencies—especially during a pandemic—it was much more likely that states would abandon their own efforts in favor of EN Express.

This was a public health tool designed by the private sector. But the private sector is not a public health authority with public health interests; their vantage points are very different.

Google and Apple imposed numerous privacy restrictions on all GAEN-based apps. Beyond the requirements for user control, the companies required that user data cannot be used for anything beyond contact tracing, including quarantine enforcement. Personal information can only be shared with a third party with user consent. But in addition to these safeguards for user data, the broader policy discussion regarding the role for contact-tracing apps in a free society needs to include other factors.

First and foremost, apps must protect user safety. As we've seen, exposure-notification apps come with a high false positive rate for exposure—and likely high false negative rates as well. High false negative rates provide users with a false sense of safety, while high false positive rates have differential impacts on various demographics. An app that unnecessarily causes someone to isolate and lose a paycheck—and possibly a job—is an app that is *not* protecting that person's health and well-being or their safety.[6]

Second, use of an exposure-notification app as a public health tool should *always be at the user's choice*. No one's access to a public site or use of a public benefit, such as voting, should ever depend on using the app. The same goes for access to private sites, including places of employment, stores, theaters, and stadiums. Australia's Privacy Amendment (Public Health Contact Information) Act 2020 guarantees that. An app can only approximate the risk that someone may be ill; if those who control a site want to prevent actual exposure from those with the virus, they must provide testing and personal protective equipment. That's the only way to know if someone is actually infected with COVID-19.[7]

Third, use of app data for any purpose other than COVID-19 proximity checking should be prohibited by law. As Google and Apple were well aware, contact-tracing apps collect information that is potentially very privacy-invasive. The companies designed the architecture to prevent data leaks, but anyone in possession of Bobby or Aliyah's phones can use the apps to learn of their encounters. Switzerland's Epidemic Act prohibits anyone from using SwissCovid data for any purposes other than informing a user that they have been in close contact with an infected person. Australia's 2020 Act does the same.[8]

Fourth, public health apps need to be evaluated both prior to deployment and during use. Testing should include how well the app integrates with existing public health infrastructure. Apps are tools of public health. Do they improve an inequitable health care situation, or make it worse? Some populations will have limited access to the apps. How does the app work in different communities? Deploying an app that lowers a given community's R_0 for a particular disease but increases other health risks is, at best, shortsighted. And, as noted in chapter 5, the app's efficacy must be continually evaluated. Data at the beginning of a given app's use reflects the app's effectiveness at that moment. As people's situations change during an epidemic, so too will their use of an app.

Fifth, policymakers should demand transparency in order to ascertain that the apps operate as promised. That means that app software should be open source. A number already are, including Singapore's TraceTogether, Germany's Corona App, and Ireland's COVID Tracker.[9]

It might be useful to institute a formal, independent testing program for apps. So far, various contact-tracing apps have had leaks and bugs. At one point, Aarogya Setu leaked the location data of some anonymized users to Google. An error in the implementation of the NHS COVID app meant that it required people to be close to infected people five times longer than necessary in order to receive an exposure notification. Google and Apple already test apps for compliance with the GAEN requirements, but by increasing transparency and providing rigor, an independent testing program would increase public trust in the apps.[10]

Though the GAEN infrastructure restricts how the apps function, the companies can't fully ensure compliance. Google and Apple aren't in a position to prevent law enforcement from acquiring proximity information from a public health agency; only a law can prevent such an event from occurring. As we have seen, though, in other instances of government surveillance, such a law would need to provide for public oversight and transparency.[11]

Only governments are in a position to control how contact-tracing apps can be used. First, though, we have to decide what we want.[12]

To better understand the trade-offs between public safety and personal privacy, it's instructive to look at how two very different entities handled the issues: South Korea and Harvard University. Both responded swiftly to the challenges posed by COVID-19. Their basic strategies—test, trace, and isolate—were the same. Their use of digital contact-tracing tools, however, were markedly different.

South Korea embarked on an aggressive contact-tracing effort using cell tower records, CCTV, and credit card records, while Harvard experimented with a Wi-Fi exposure notification tool that it quickly abandoned. The Asian nation and the elite university shared a clear sense of where they stood on issues of privacy and public safety. Both had long debated the appropriate balance between public safety and digital privacy. It's worth looking briefly at how they got there.

Recall the South Korean experience with MERS. By all accounts, South Korea handled the outbreak badly. By the time the index patient was diagnosed, he had infected twenty-eight people, two of whom infected another 109. All but two of these infections occurred in hospitals, where the infected patient hadn't been isolated from others (including in the waiting room). Test, trace, and isolate didn't happen until it was much too late. Nor did the government let people know where infections were occurring.[13]

In 2020, South Korea was determined not to repeat its previous failure. After MERS, the nation put the right services in place for the next epidemic—for there would surely be another. Korea's first step was to ensure that diagnostic tests would be readily available. The government invested in companies that developed diagnostic technologies while modifying regulations to ensure that, in the event of an outbreak of a new infectious disease, new diagnostic tests would be rapidly approved. When COVID-19 hit, this groundwork made a huge difference. Five weeks after its first COVID-19 case, Korea could run 15,000 tests per day.[14]

A functional contact-tracing system requires that public health authorities can quickly determine where an infected person has been and locate their close contacts. Korea opted to use cell tower and credit card records to speed up the work of manual contact tracers. A decade ago, it would have been a violation of privacy laws for public health authorities to do this. Korea's 2011 Personal Information Protection Act bans the collection, use, and disclosure of personal data without an individual's consent. In 2015, however, after the crisis of MERS, Korea amended its Infectious Disease Control and Prevention Act to allow the Ministry of Health and Welfare (MOHW) and the Korea Centers for Disease Control and Prevention (KCDC) to rapidly access cell tower and credit card records in the event of an infectious outbreak.[15]

Not every choice that Korea made worked out well. In some cases, the release of details on where infected people had traveled while infectious proved problematic. The amended Infectious Disease Control and Prevention Act gave MOHW access to a lot of information about an infected person: age, nationality, gender, location (including from their cell phones), transit pass records—and more. MOHW then posted a daily report on the age, nationality, gender and locations of infected people. Some local governments went further, publishing the names of restaurants, churches, and shops visited by the infected people. Inevitably, Internet trolls played detective, identifying and harassing some of the infected individuals. Some were stigmatized, accused of having affairs, paying for sex, or cheating on insurance.[16]

After several such incidents, Korea's public health agencies decided to publish less information about the infected individuals, making it more difficult for others to identify them (for some, of course, the damage had already been done). Yet the underlying choices Korea had made about trade-offs between public health and personal privacy proved popular—even though not all the initial actions were appropriate.[17]

As with Korea, Harvard's decisions on digital contact tracing built on top of an earlier failure. In 2012, after a press story about widespread cheating in "Introduction to Congress," an undergraduate government course, Harvard administrators authorized a search of emails of college resident deans to find out if any had leaked news of the scandal to the press (resident deans live in Harvard residential houses, advise students, and teach courses). The residential deans learned of the search only months later. That the search was just of email headers did little to mitigate their consternation. Much soul searching—and a new policy on access to electronic information—followed.[18]

The new policy made clear to everyone at Harvard—staff, students, and faculty—that their electronic communications were considered private. The university could only access a user's electronic information—emails, voice mails, text messages, as well as tracks of Internet usage and logs of access to facilities—for "legitimate and important" purposes. This access had to be limited in scope, with clear records to ensure compliance with university policy. Aside from routine system protection, maintenance, and management, access would be only with the permission of a dean or senior administrator; afterwards cases are subject to review by an oversight committee.[19]

With this policy, Harvard made a strong and public commitment to privacy. That approach governed the university's development of TraceFi, the Wi-Fi–based exposure notification system the university piloted in the summer of 2020. The university had instituted a rigorous COVID-19 testing regime, requiring testing three days per week for staff, students, and faculty living on campus and two days per week for those on campus more than once a week or having high contact with students. Harvard, in other words, implemented test, trace, and isolate as well as smartphone-based proximity exposure notifications. With this system of frequent testing in place, TraceFi wasn't turning up new cases. Once you've decided that access to electronic information must be only for "legitimate and important" purposes, a surveillance system that isn't efficacious just doesn't cut it. TraceFi didn't last past its pilot test.[20]

Some commentators find Korea's surveillance excessive. Certainly some of the data collected—cell site location, credit-card information—violates user consent, while some of the state's other actions—publication of routes of infected people—have harmed individuals. Others argue that not every institution can afford a testing regimen as robust as Harvard's. The point, though, is that both South Korea and Harvard had serious policy discussions about the trade-offs between public safety and digital privacy before the crisis hit. The decisions they made in response to COVID-19 were in accordance with their earlier choices.

Proximity-based contact-tracing apps represent an enormous social experiment, one that has the potential to change the nature of our interactions. Brief encounters, unscheduled and unexpected, have been ephemeral parts of our lives for most of human existence. The knowledge of these interactions, and whether we spent two minutes—or ten—chatting by the coffee machine, was ours alone. Proximity-checking apps upend that. Instead of informal encounters that remain only in the minds of the individuals involved, we will have created an electronic record. Knowing that records of these encounters exist changes how we think about them.

We behave differently when we know our actions are recorded—even if we're the only ones who have access to the data. We'll inevitably change how we interact, and something immeasurable will be lost. And once we've used these apps for a while, we'll start thinking about the collection of such information as normal. It will seem only natural to have this information available during emergencies.

One worry, of course, is mission creep. The current GAEN-based system—both the infrastructure and the apps themselves—was designed to reveal exposure without disclosing through whom, when, or where the exposure occurred. But if we've normalized the idea of collecting proximity data, the idea that such data could be used to make us feel safe from bad things—criminals, terrorists, kidnappers—might not seem so outlandish. Investigators already use "cell tower dumps" to find bank robbers and other criminals. Repressive governments, immigration authorities, and law enforcement agencies could use proximity data to track political opponents, immigrants, activists—or government leakers.[21]

One has only to reflect on the 9/11 attacks to recall how rapidly surveillance powers can expand during an emergency. Five years after the terrorist attacks, Americans learned that the government was warrantlessly wiretapping their communications from abroad and collecting domestic call records—who phoned whom, when, and for how long—in bulk, in the absence of any law explicitly authorizing that collection. The use of proximity-based contact-tracing apps conditions us to accept that it is normal for electronic devices to track our contacts. With time, we may see such apps becoming the norm outside a pandemic. That would be a dangerous situation indeed.

A 1993 National Academies study on the social impact of AIDS observed, "An epidemic is both a medical and social occurrence." This observation takes our study back to where we began: the medical aspects of COVID-19. The pandemic revealed to the public at large a phenomenon that has been obvious to public health authorities for decades: the United States is two societies when it comes to health, separate but unequal. Discriminatory policies have led to marginalized populations living in less healthy environments, having less access to health care, and having poorer health outcomes. COVID-19 has produced a vastly higher rate of infections and deaths in low-income and non-white populations in the United States, a pattern that has been repeated in the UK, France, and elsewhere.[22]

Contact-tracing apps can be effective only if people believe they are safe to use. The apps are, as the actor Stewart Reynolds put it in a video on the Canadian app, a "supersimple" way for you to find out if you've been exposed to a confirmed case of COVID-19 and "get checked, stay healthy, and protect your friends and loved ones." But you can't stay healthy and protect your friends and loved ones without a public health infrastructure to support you. Without robust laws that prevent law enforcement and immigration officials from accessing the information collected by proximity-checking apps, and without a social infrastructure that supports people when they must stay home from work, contact-tracing apps are of limited value to the marginalized populations who need them the most. And they are of no help at all to people who don't have the requisite smartphones—or who lack the digital literacy to use the apps.[23]

What we need to know about a contact-tracing app is: Is it efficacious? Does the app help or hinder the efforts of human-based contact tracing, a practice central to ending epidemics? If not—and efficacy must be measured across different communities—there is no reason to consider its use any further. Is the use of the app equitable? What are the social and legal protections for people who receive an exposure notification? Does a contact-tracing app improve public health more effectively than other efforts? Does the public support its use? Without public support, apps fail.

For apps to be widely adopted and really have an impact, we need an equitable public health system, one that makes people confident they will be cared for if they fall ill. We need that as well as strong and protective laws that keep public health information with public health officials. Only then might marginalized populations be willing to trust contact tracing, whether conducted by humans or apps, and act on the information they provide.

At some point, the COVID-19 pandemic will end, but inevitably, another one will appear. The next one will almost certainly be different from COVID-19, but whatever it is, it will still be dangerous. Pandemics kill people. Now is the time to decide what sorts of medical and social interventions we will make and what choices we want. Now is the time to create the medical and social infrastructure that supports whatever decision we make. The choices we make now will reverberate forever.

ACKNOWLEDGMENTS

In late March 2020, Greg Nojeim of the Center for Democracy and Technology (CDT) organized a task force with members from tech companies, academia, health care, and civil liberties organizations to look at the issues of privacy and user data in the time of COVID-19. Our first discussion on location motivated me to write a blog post on efficacy of the use of location data. Our semi-weekly meetings have been thought-provoking and provided many insights reflected in these pages. I am very grateful to Greg and the folks at CDT.

My first two blog posts on COVID-19 were on efficacy of contact-tracing apps; my third, with Christy Lopez and Laura Moy, focused on contact-tracing apps and equity issues. Little did we know as we put together our post in late April how these concerns would become a national priority shortly afterwards. I learned much from Christy and Laura—and continue to do so. The post we wrote provided the inspiration for this book.

I owe thanks to the National Science Foundation. Funding for a related project on the use of communications metadata not only led to academic research that I have published elsewhere, but also influenced ideas that are reflected here.

I came at this project with a background of computer science, specifically, in communications surveillance and privacy. I needed to understand the public health issues, and that meant talking with those in the trenches. I needed to learn how to do that. My conversation with and readings from Barbara Grosz helped me understand what I needed to ask the contact tracers and other health professionals with whom I spoke. Those were invaluable lessons.

To say that COVID-19 has made it an extremely busy time for those in public health is to engage in the opposite of hyperbole; no words can really capture what time has been like for epidemiologists, contact tracers, and others handling the medical side of the crisis. I am particularly grateful to Bill Darrow, David Heymann, Bryant Karras, Shefali Oza, Marcel Salathé, Josh Scharfstein, and Jonathan Zenilman, who took time out of an extraordinarily hectic period to talk with me. I am also extremely grateful to Dick Conlon, Terry Cullen, Beth Meyerson, John Potterat, Rich Rothenberg, and Ryane Sickles, who educated me about the human kind of contact tracers. My neighbor, John Urshel, who works at Partners in Health, connected me to contact tracers in Liberia, and I owe thanks to him and his Partners in Health colleague Viola Karanja for doing so. Garmai Cyrus, Lassana Jabteh, and Willis Archie Yasnine of Partners in Health took time from COVID-19 contact tracing in Liberia to talk with me about Ebola contact tracing, answering my innumerable questions; I am extremely grateful. Others, including Zinzi Bailey and Nicole Triplett, answered questions I didn't know I had. Such education is extremely valuable.

My academic home is in cybersecurity policy, and my long-time colleagues Bart Preneel and Ron Rivest explained some of the background thinking involved in the apps used in the GAEN effort. Stefano Tessaro and Carmela Troncoso were particularly generous with their time and thoughts. I am also grateful to Steve Bellovin, Mark Brier, Pam Dixon, Lilian Edwards, Stu

Feldman, Urs Gasser, Constantine Gatsonis, Benoit Gaucherin, Giles Hogben, Dennis Jackson, John Langford, Doug Leith, Sue Moon, K. S. Park, and Jim Waldo, all of whom provided very useful information on a variety of topics. I also appreciate the help of Raman Jit Singh Chima, Lalitesh Katragadda, Srinvas Kodali, Smitha Krishna Prasad, and Rahul Matthan for filling me in on Aarogya Setu. As I began this project, my questions were imprecise and libraries were closed. Natalia Espinosa researched background material despite these challenges, and I am grateful to her for the help she provided.

My readers—Jon Callas, Mark Donner, Susan Ernst, Sharon Bradford Franklin, and Nicole Triplett—made numerous insightful points, pressed me hard on issues that needed clarification, and corrected errors. They provided extremely useful guidance, and they did so on a remarkably tight timetable. I feel extremely lucky for their kind and generous help. Any remaining errors are mine, of course.

I worked with Audra Wolfe on my previous book, *Listening In: Cybersecurity in an Insecure Age*. There she helped transform my technologist's thoughts into a flowing narrative with words that sometimes soared. *People Count*, with its tales of epidemiologists and computer scientists, pandemics and smartphones, provided significantly more of a challenge—and on a very tight timetable. Audra again worked her magic, helping me to hone my thinking and my writing, enabling this ambitious project to come to fruition. She did this with remarkable patience and energy despite my growing lateness on chapters. This book would not have been completed without her help; I cannot thank her enough.

My first reader and strongest booster is my husband Neil. Early on in COVID we acquired a new puppy, which was both a welcome distraction as well as companion for Neil while I disappeared into my study to write this book. I look forward to now returning to a version of normal life that includes hikes on the weekends, dinners that take longer than a rushed twenty minutes, and conversations that are not solely about how to interweave the ideas I've just considered into the text. I also can't wait to be gathering with friends and family, teaching in front of a classroom of actual students—and not their Zoom embodiments—and seeing theater and ballet in person. That might yet take time, but how grand it will be when we get there.

NOTES

Preface

1. "In mid-February some": Encryption Working Group, Carnegie Endowment for International Peace, *Moving the Encryption Policy Conversation Forward*, September 2019, https://carnegieendowment.org/2019/09/10/moving-encryption-policy-conversation-forward-pub-79573.

2. "I was also": This was the RSA meeting, https://www.rsaconference.com/about/press-releases/rsa-conference-2020-kicks-off-in-san-francisco.

3. "Two weeks later": Roni Caryn Rabin, "Lost Sense of Smell May Be Peculiar Clue to Coronavirus Infection," *New York Times*, March 22, 2020.

4. "'Google Searches Can'": Seth Stephens-Davidowitz, "Google Searches Can Help Us Find Emerging COVID-19 Outbreaks," *New York Times*, April 5, 2020. "One has to": David Lazer and Ryan Kennedy, "What We Can Learn about the Epic Failure of Google Flu Trends," *Wired*, October 1, 2015, and Yunyun Zhou et al., "Lost Sense of Smell May Be Peculiar Clue to Coronavirus Infection," *Opthalmology* 127, no. 7 (July 2020): 982–983.

5. "At just the": Susan Landau, "Categorizing Uses of Communications Metadata: Systematizing Knowledge and Presenting a Path for Privacy," *New Security Paradigms Workshop*, 2020. "Meanwhile, I was": Susan Landau, "Location Surveillance to Counter COVID-19: Efficacy Is What Matters," *Lawfare*, March 25, 2020, https://www.lawfareblog.com/looking-beyond-contact-tracing-stop-spread. "As I learned": Susan Landau, "Looking beyond Contact Tracing to Stop the Spread," *Lawfare*, April 10, 2020, https://www.lawfareblog.com/location-surveillance-counter-covid-19-efficacy-what-matters. "Then, along with": Susan Landau, Christy Lopez, and

Laura Moy, "The Importance of Equity in Contact Tracing," *Lawfare*, May 1, 2020, https://www.lawfareblog.com/importance-equity-contact-tracing.

Chapter 1

1. "As a science": "Microbiology by Numbers," *Nature Reviews Microbiology* 9, no. 628 (2011), https://doi.org/10.1038/nrmicro2644.

2. "His experiment showed": Paula Gottdenker, "Francesco Redi and the Fly Experiments," *Bulletin of the History of Medicine* 53, no. 4 (Winter 1979): 575–592.

3. "Snow didn't buy": John Snow, *On the Mode of Communication of Cholera* (London: John Churchill, 1849), 11–23.

4. "What Snow had": ibid., 5. "Snow posited that": ibid., 8–9, 20–21. "He began studying": Snow, *On the Mode of Communication of Cholera*, 2nd ed. (London: John Churchill, 1855), 38–39.

5. "Snow quickly realized," "He collected drinking," and "Later samples had": ibid., 39. "Snow did not": Steven Johnson, *The Ghost Map: The Story of London's Most Terrifying Epidemic—And How It Changed Science, Cities, and the Modern World* (New York: Riverhead Books, 2006), 140–143.

6. "When he infected": Paul de Kruif, *Microbe Hunters* (New York: Harcourt, Brace, 1996), 104–115.

7. "The history of": Arthur Albert St. Mouritz, *The Flu: A Brief History of Influenza in U.S. America, Europe, Hawaii* (Honolulu, HI: Advertiser Publishing, 1921), 7, and W. I. B. Beveridge, "The Chronicle of Influenza Epidemics," *History and Philosophy of the Life Sciences* 13, no. 2 (1991): 224–225. "Long before airplanes": ibid., 225. "Relatively accurate records": M. E. Kitler, P. Gavino, and D. Lavanchy, "Influenza and the Work of the World Health Organization," *Vaccine* 20 (2002): 7, and Beveridge, "Chronicle of Influenza Epidemics," 225.

8. "But over the": "How the Flu Virus Can Change: 'Drift' and 'Shift,'" Centers for Disease Control and Prevention, https://www.cdc.gov/flu/about/viruses/change.htm.

9. "When new versions": S.-E. Mamelund, "Influenza, Historical," in *International Encyclopedia of Public Health*, vol. 3, ed. Kris Heggenhouggen and Stella Quah (San Diego: Academic Press, 2008), 597–609.

10. "Although the *Yersinia*": "Plague," World Health Organization, https://www.who.int/ith/diseases/plague/en.

11. "R_0 estimates for": Steven Sanche et al., "High Contagiousness and Rapid Spread of Severe Acute Respiratory Syndrome Coronavirus 2," *Emerging Infectious Diseases* 26, no. 7 (July 2020). "With better data": Sam Abbott et al., "The Transmissibility of Novel Coronavirus in the Early Stages of the 2019–20 Outbreak in Wuhan: Exploring Initial Point-Source Exposure Sizes and Durations Using Scenario Analysis," *Wellcome Open Research* 5, no. 17 (2020), https://doi.org/10.12688/wellcomeopenres.15718.1.

12. "The R_0 for": In locations where vaccination is prevalent, measles is a childhood disease because everyone else has immunity either through having had the disease or through vaccination. See Sheldon G. Cohen, "Measles and Immunodulation," *The Journal of Allergy and Clinical Immunology* 121 (February 2008): 543. "Smallpox has a": Centers for Disease Control and Prevention, "Measles" (April 15, 2019). "Yet the Spanish": Centers for Disease Control and Prevention, "1918 Pandemic (H1N1 virus)" (March 20, 2019), https://www.cdc.gov/flu/pandemic-resources/1918-pandemic-h1n1.html.

13. "A classic example": World Health Organization, *Global Tuberculosis Report* (Geneva: World Health Organization, 2018), 1.

14. "The leading US": Berkeley Lovelace Jr., "Dr. Anthony Fauci Says Coronavirus Turned 'Out to Be My Worst Nightmare' and It 'Isn't Over,'" CNBC, June 9, 2020.

15. "We don't know": Frank Fenner et al., *Smallpox*, History of International Public Health, no. 6 (Geneva: World Health Organization, 1988), 211.

16. "Highly contagious and": Fenner et al., *Smallpox*, 229. "The epidemics that": Noble David Cook and W. George Lovell, eds., *Secret Judgments of God: Old World Disease in Colonial Spanish America, The Civilization of the American Indian Series* (Norman: University of Oklahoma Press, 1992).

17. "Thanks to several": Not everyone agrees, as there are vials of the disease at the US Centers for Disease Control and Prevention and at Vector, a virology lab in Siberia. The vials are highly protected, but there is much concern over retaining smallpox anywhere. Smallpox would be an extremely effective biological weapon given the world's lack of immunity. "Vaccination against smallpox": It appears that variolation originated in China or India.

Arthur Bolyston, "The Origins of Inoculation," *Journal of the Royal Society of Medicine* 105, no. 5 (July 2012): 309–313.

18. "Instead, by the": Fenner et al., *Smallpox*, 216.

19. "That this even": Fenner et al., *Smallpox*, 171–172. "In Europe, Canada": The information on Europe and the US is from ibid., 317. From the same book, we learn about Canada, 332–333; Mexico, 335; the remaining nations in Central America, 327 and 329; and South America, 335. "In 1959 the": ibid., 394–395.

20. "Studies in Pakistan": Fenner et al., *Smallpox*, 481.

21. "Prior to the": Fenner et al., *Smallpox*, 476. "The patients hadn't": William H. Foege, *House on Fire: The Fight to Eradicate Smallpox* (Berkeley: University of California Press, 2011), 114.

22. "The strategy worked": Fenner et al., *Smallpox*, 1062–1063. This was the last "naturally occurring" case; there were also a few cases from lab accidents.

23. "In this case": Stephen D. Lawn and Zumla Alimudden, "Tuberculosis," *Lancet* 378, no. 9785 (2011): 57–72. "Today, TB kills": World Health Organization, "Tuberculosis," https://www.who.int/news-room/fact-sheets/detail/tuberculosis.

24. "Since there was": Judith Walzer Leavitt, *Typhoid Mary: Captive to the Public Health* (Boston: Beacon Press, 1996). "When there is": ibid., 57, 255.

25. "Contact tracing also": Emily Gurley, "Balancing Public Good with Privacy, Autonomy, and Confidentiality," https://www.coursera.org/learn/covid-19-contact-tracing?edocomorp=covid-19-contact-tracing. "The questions a": John J. Potterat, *Seeking the Positives: A Life Spent on the Cutting Edge of Public Health* (self-published, 2015), 5.

Chapter 2

1. "The authorities first": Derrick Tovey, "The Bradford Smallpox Outbreak in 1962: A Personal Account," *Journal of the Royal Society of Medicine* 97, no. 5 (2004): 244–247, https://doi.org/10.1177/014107680409700512.

2. "The hematologist, Derrick": Tovey, "Bradford Smallpox Outbreak."

3. "Tovey turned to": Tovey, "Bradford Smallpox Outbreak."

4. "She had emigrated": Eric Butterworth, "The 1962 Smallpox Outbreak and the British Press," *Race* 7, no. 4 (April 1966): 349, https://doi.org/10.1177/030639686600700403. "When the child": Frank Fenner et al., *Smallpox and Its Eradication*, History of International Public Health, no. 6 (Geneva: World Health Organization, 1988), 1079.

5. "The girl had": J. Douglas and W. Edgar, "Smallpox in Bradford, 1962," *British Medical Journal* 1, no. 5278 (1962): 612–614, https://doi.org/10.1136/bmj.1.5278.612. "The delay in": Tovey, "Bradford Smallpox Outbreak." "A potential 1,400": Fenner et al., *Smallpox*, 1079. "Even with the": Douglas and Edgar, "Smallpox in Bradford, 1962." "The British public": Michael Dwyer and Gareth Millward, "Vaccinating Britain: Mass Vaccination and the Public since the Second World War," *Social History of Medicine* 33, no. 1 (February 2020): 344–346, https://doi.org/10.1093/shm/hkz087. "Within five days": Fenner et al., *Smallpox*, 1079.

6. "Just two months": Fenner et al., *Smallpox*, 324 and 332.

7. "In contrast to": William H. Foege, *House on Fire: The Fight to Eradicate Smallpox* (Berkeley: University of California Press, 2011), 21.

8. "The baby was": Foege, *House on Fire*, 21–22.

9. "The complexity of": World Health Organization, "Pneumonia of Unknown Cause—China" (January 5, 2020), https://www.who.int/csr/don/05-january-2020-pneumonia-of-unkown-cause-china/en/. "By mid-January 2020": Chaolin Huang et al., "Clinical Features of Patients Infected with 2019 Novel Coronavirus in Wuhan, China," *Lancet* 395, no. 10223 (2020): 497–506. "In mid-March, people" and "More symptoms have": Roni Caryn Rabin, "Lost Sense of Smell May Be Peculiar Clue to Coronavirus Infection," *New York Times*, March 22, 2020.

10. "There's something else": Roberta Bivens, "'The People Have No More Left for the Commonwealth': Media, Migration, and Identity in the 1961–1962 British Smallpox Outbreak," *Immigration and Minorities* 25, no. 3 (November 2007): 263–289. "A small manufacturing": Butterworth, "The 1962 Smallpox Outbreak," 348. "Days before the": "Keep Out the Germs," *Daily Mail*, January 3, 1962. "When smallpox was": Tovey, "Bradford Smallpox Outbreak," and Butterworth, "The 1962 Smallpox Outbreak."

11. "This sore usually": This can happen when kissing an infected person who has an open mouth sore.

12. "Mercury is toxic": John Frith, "Syphilis—Its Early History and Treatment until Penicillin and the Debate on Its Origins," *Journal of Military and Veterans' Health* 20, no. 4 (November 2012). "But the ghostlike": Hendrik Ibsen's play *Ghosts* presents a searing and bleak view of the consequences of untreated syphilis.

13. "The result was": Albert Gallatin Love and Charles Benedict Davenport, "Defects Found in Drafted Men: Statistical Information Compiled from the Draft Records Showing the Physical Condition of the Men Registered and Examined in Pursuance of the Requirements of the Selective-Service Act" (U.S. Government Printing Office, 1920), 84. "Putting young men": Allan M. Brandt, *No Magic Bullet: A Social History of Venereal Disease in the United States since 1880, with a New Chapter on AIDS* (Oxford: Oxford University Press, 1987), 115 and fn. 70. "By the 1930s": Parran writes that 683,000 Americans were under treatment or observation for syphilis in 1935; this was out of an estimated population of 127 million. Thomas Parran, *Shadow on the Land: Syphilis* (New York: Reynal and Hitchcock, 1937), 54. "Sexually transmitted diseases": Elizabeth Gettleman and Mark Murrmann, "The Enemy in Your Pants: The Military's Decades-Long War against STDs," *Mother Jones* (May–June 2010), accessed July 6, 2020, https://www.motherjones.com/media/2010/05/us-military-std-posters/.

14. "This was an": James Jones, who wrote about the Tuskegee study, described PHS effort as "cover[ing] the nation with a Wasserman dragnet. The campaign reached whites and blacks alike. . . ." James H. Jones, *Bad Blood: The Tuskegee Syphilis Experiment*, new and expanded edition (New York: Free Press, 1993), 89. "In Macon County": Susan M. Reverby, *Examining Tuskegee: The Infamous Syphilis Study and Its Legacy* (Chapel Hill: University of North Carolina Press, 2009), 62.

15. "A study conducted": E. Bruusgaard, "Über das Schicksal der nicht spezifisch behaldeelten Luetiker," *Archive für Dermatologie und Syphilis* 157 (1929): 309–332. "So, Clark proposed": Jones, *Bad Blood*, 93.

16. "Reports of the": Allan M. Brandt, *Racism and Research: The Case of the Tuskegee Syphilis Study*, Hastings Center Report 8, 21. "Local physicians knew": Jones, *Bad Blood*, 144–145. "When World War": Jones, *Bad Blood*, 177–178. "Only after an": Jean Heller, "Syphilis Victims in U.S. Study Went Untreated for 40 Years," *New York Times*, July 26, 1972. "Somewhere

between 28": Brandt, "Racism and Research," 21–29; see also endnote 1 of the Brandt paper.

17. "On the one": Jones, *Bad Blood*, 41.

18. "It sowed mistrust" and "Middle-aged and older": Marcella Alsan and Marianne Wannamaker, "Tuskegee and the Health of Black Men," *Quarterly Journal of Economics* 133, no. 1 (February 2018): 407–455. "More broadly, it": Brian D. Smedley, Adrienne Y. Stith, and Alan R. Nelson, eds., *Unequal Treatment: Confronting Racial and Ethnic Disparities in Health Care* (Washington, DC: National Academies Press, 2003), 5.

19. "The contact-tracing portion": Syphilis testing is the underlying reason for premarital blood tests; the testing, however, has high false positive rates. It also doesn't work as well as intended, since premarital sex is quite common. "These workers were": Beth E. Meyerson, Fred A. Martich and Gerald Naehr, *Ready to Go: The History and Contributions of U.S. Public Health Advisors* (Research Triangle Park, NC: American Social Health Association, 2008), 87. "They needed an" and "And because it": ibid., 60.

20. "Their role was": Richard T. Conlon, *From the Merry Widow Bar To . . . : Tales of a Venereal Disease Investigator during the 1960s and 1970s* (self-published, 2019), 27.

21. "They began by" and "Then the contact": Mary Chamberland and William Darrow, "The Early Years of AIDS: CDC's Response to a Historic Epidemic," *The Global Health Chronicles* (2016): 17:25–17:33, https://www.globalhealthchronicles.org/items/show/6870.

22. "PHAs practiced role": Conlon, *From the Merry Widow*, 20. "Often another try": ibid., 28–29.

23. "When the PHA": Meyerson et al., *Ready to Go*, 133.

24. "Even so, and": Conlon, *From the Merry Widow*, 71. "I'd go in": Richard Conlon (Public Health Advisor, retired), interview with the author, July 1, 2020.

25. "But when Conlon": Conlon, personal communication, July 21, 2020.

26. "In the 1940s": This figure was calculated on the basis that 0.7 percent of white deaths and 3.1 percent of non-white deaths were due to syphilis. Harold A. Kahn and Albert P. Iskrant, "Syphilis Mortality Analysis 1933–45," *Journal of Venereal Disease Information* 29–30 (July 1948):

193. In 1940, the white population was 89.8 percent and the Black population was 9.8 percent of the total. US Census Bureau, "A Look at the 1940 Census," 9, https://www.census.gov/newsroom/cspan/1940census /CSPAN_1940slides.pdf. "The work of": Meyerson et al., *Ready to Go*, 146.

27. "In 1980 an": Randy Shilts, *And the Band Played On: Politics, People, and the AIDS Epidemic* (New York: St. Martin's Griffin, 1988), 39. "The results were": ibid., 42–43. "In early 1981": ibid., 55. "Then a Haitian": ibid., 56, and Mary Chamberland and Mary Guinan, *The Early Years of AIDS: CDC's Response to a Historic Epidemic*. The Global Health Chronicles, 2016, https://www.globalhealthchronicles.org/items/show/5393 22:00–24:05. "Later in the": Shilts, *And the Band Played On*, 60. "More cases of": "Pneumocystis Pneumonia—Los Angeles," *Morbidity and Mortality Weekly Report* 30, no. 21 (June 5, 1981): 1–3.

28. "At this point": Shilts, *And the Band Played On*, 66. "She became convinced": ibid., 83. "Back at the": ibid., 88.

29. "On that basis": Centers for Disease Control and Prevention, "Current Trends Prevention of Acquired Immune Deficiency Syndrome (AIDS): Report of Inter-Agency Recommendations," *Morbidity and Mortality Weekly Report* 32, no. 8 (March 4, 1983). "DNA studies later": M. Thomas P. Gilbert et al., "The Emergence of HIV/AIDS in the Americas and Beyond," *Proceedings of the National Academies of Science* 104, no. 47 (2007): 18566–18570.

30. "Studies had shown": H. W. Jaffe et al., "National Case Control Study of Kaposi's Sarcoma and Pneumocystis carinii Pneumonia in Homosexual Men: Epidemiologic Results," *Annals of Internal Medicine* 99 (1983): 145–151.

31. "He added, 'For'": John J. Potterat (Director STD/AIDS Program, El Paso County Department of Health and Environment, Colorado Springs, retired), personal communication, July 22, 2020.

32. "We can contact": Potterat, personal communication, July 22, 2020.

33. "Beginning in 1986": J. Stan Lehman, Simone C. Gray, and Jonathan H. Mermin, "Prevalence and Public Health Implications of State Laws That Criminalize Potential HIV Exposure in the United States," *AIDS Behavior* 18, no. 6 (2014): 997–1006. "In some states": Sergio Hernandez, "Sex, Lies, and HIV: What You Don't Tell Your Partner Is a Crime," ProPublica (December 1, 2013).

34. "It would start" and "The discussion would": Ryane Sickels (HIV Intervention Specialist), interview with the author, July 8, 2020.

35. "'I want to'": Sickels, interview with the author, July 8, 2020.

36. "Their role cannot": John J. Potterat, *Seeking the Positives: A Life Spent on the Cutting Edge of Public Health* (self-published, 2015), 7.

37. "In the first": Centers for Disease Control and Prevention, "Update: Acquired Immunodeficiency Syndrome—United States," *Morbidity and Mortality Weekly Report* 35 (January 17, 1986). "The PHAs had": Meyerson et al., *Ready to Go*, 112–116. "Women were not": ibid., 117–123. "And until the": Beth Meyerson (Research Professor, Southwest Institute for Research on Women, University of Arizona), interview with the author, July 1, 2020.

38. "Black Americans make": "What Is the Impact of HIV on Racial and Ethnic Minorities in the U.S.?" (HIV.gov, June 18, 2020), https://www.hiv .gov/hiv-basics/overview/data-and-trends/impact-on-racial-and-ethnic -minorities.

39. "The two groups": Meyerson, interview with the author, July 1, 2020. "But understanding what": A. S. Klovdahl et al., "Social Networks and Infectious Disease: The Colorado Springs Study," *Social Science and Medicine* 38, no. 1 (1994): 79–88.

40. "The disease is": Xiaver Pourrut et al., "The Natural History of the Ebola Virus in Africa," *Microbes and Infection* 7 (2005): 1006.

41. "There is no": There is no Ebola treatment drug licensed in the US; two experimental drugs that were used in a 2018 outbreak in eastern Congo had good results. See National Institutes of Health, "Two Drugs Reduce Risk of Death from Ebola" (December 10, 2019), https://www.nih.gov/news -events/nih-research-matters/two-drugs-reduce-risk-death-ebola.

42. "Ebola first emerged": Pourrut et al., "Natural History." "Most outbreaks have": Centers for Disease Control and Prevention, "Ebola Virus Distribution Map: Cases of Ebola Virus Disease in Africa since 1976" (June 19, 2019), https://www.cdc.gov/vhf/ebola/history/distribution-map.html, and Centers for Disease Control and Prevention, "2014–2016 Ebola Outbreak Distribution in West Africa" (March 18, 2019), https://www.cdc.gov /vhf/ebola/history/2014-2016-outbreak/distribution-map.html. These are the official records on number of deaths; it is believed that many deaths went unrecorded.

43. "The earlier outbreaks": Medicins Sans Frontieres, "Pushed to the Limit and Beyond: A Year into the Largest Ever Ebola Outbreak" (2015), 6. The disease was apparently spreading in Sierra Leone for five months before it was discovered; see Cordelia Coltart et al., "The Ebola Outbreak, 2013–2016: Old Lessons for New Epidemics," *Philosophical Transactions Royal Society London B. Biological Science* 372 (May 26, 2017).

44. "Quarantine orders such": Preeti Emrick, Christine Gentry, and Lauren Morowit, "Ebola Virus Disease: International Perspective on Enhanced Health Surveillance, Disposition of the Dead, and Their Effect on Isolation and Quarantine Practices," *Disaster and Military Medicine* 2 (2016).

45. "Infected people were" and "The centers were": Samuel Cohn and Ruth Kutalek, "Historical Parallels, Ebola Virus Disease and Cholera: Understanding Community Distrust and Social Violence with Epidemics," *PLOS Current* 8 (2016). "The policies were": "End of the Ebola Outbreak in DRC," *The Lancet Podcast* Ebola Collection, Global Health (July 17, 2019): 2:13–2:28, https://www.thelancet.com/pb-assets/Lancet/stories/audio/lancet/2018/TL_Jul_18_ebola-1532448813063.mp3.

46. "Government burial policy": Angellar Manguvo and Mafuvadze Benford, "The Impact of Traditional and Religious Practices on the Spread of Ebola in West Africa: Time for a Strategic Shift," *Pan African Medical Journal* 22, suppl. 1 (2015). "But because contact": Umberto Pellecchia et al., "Social Consequences of Ebola Containment Measures in Liberia," *PLOS One* 10, no. 12 (2015): e0143036. "A safe burial": World Health Organization, *How to Conduct Safe and Dignified Burial of a Patient Who Has Died from Suspected or Confirmed Ebola or Marburg Virus Disease, Interim Guidance* (2017).

47. "Teams working in": David L. Heymann (Professor of Infectious Disease Epidemiology, London School of Hygiene and Tropical Medicine), interview with the author, July 6, 2020.

48. "Some believed government": Robert A. Blair, Benjamin S. Morse, and Lily L. Tsai, "Public Health and Public Trust: Survey Evidence from the Ebola Virus Epidemic in Liberia," *Social Science and Medicine* 172 (2017): 90. "'Politicians and lawmakers'" and "'Communities became resistant'": Garmai Cyrus (Mental Health Counselor, Partners in Health), interview with the author, June 30, 2020.

49. "'We had to'" and "It also enabled": Willis Archie Yasnine (Mental Health Counselor, Partners in Health), interview with the author, June 30, 2020. "There was lots": Lassana Jabateh (Community Health Director, Partners in Health), interview with the author, June 30, 2020.

50. "'And the community'": Cyrus, interview with the author, June 30, 2020.

51. "A zoonotic disease": Ji-Eun Park, Soyoung Jung, Aeran Kim, and Ji-Eun Park, "MERS Transmission and Risk Factors: A Systematic Review," *BMC Public Health* 18, no. 574 (2018). "Of the 1,100": Choe Sung-Hun, "Fears of MERS Virus Prompt Broadening of Cautions in South Korea," *New York Times*, June 3, 2020.

52. "A week after": Sun Young Cho et al., "MERS-CoV Outbreak Following a Single Patient Exposure in Emergency Room in South Korea: An Epidemiological Outbreak Study," *Lancet* 388, no. 10048 (2016): 994–1001, and K. H. Kim et al., "Middle East Respiratory Syndrome Coronavirus (MERS-CoV) Outbreak in South Korea, 2015: Epidemiology, Characteristics, and Public Health Implications," *Journal of Hospital Infection* 95, no. 2 (2017). "By the time, "A total of," and "It failed to": ibid. "The biggest spread": Hiroshi Nihkiura et al., "Identifying Determinants of Heterogeneous Transmission Dynamics of the Middle East Respiratory Syndrome (MERS) Outbreak in the Republic of Korea, 2015: A Retrospective Epidemiological Analysis," *BMJ Open* 6, no. 2 (2016).

53. "When the coronavirus": Government of the Republic of Korea, *Tackling COVID-19 Health, Quarantine and Economic Measures: Korean Experience* (March 31, 2020), 11.

54. "The United States": COVID Tracking Project, US Historical Data, accessed July 9, 2020, https://covidtracking.com/data/us-daily, and David Lee and Jaehong Lee, "Testing on the Move: South Korea's Rapid Response to the COVID-10 Pandemic," *Transportation Research Interdisciplinary Perspectives* 5 (2020): 100111.

55. "Under the Infectious": This is the Contagious Disease Prevention and Control Act. Sangchul Park, Gina Jeehyun Choi, and Haksoo Ko, "Response to COVID-19 in South Korea—Privacy Controversies," *JAMA* 323, no. 21 (April 23, 2020): 2129–2130. "The location information": Hyonhee Shin, Hunjoo Jin, and Josh Smith, "How South Korea Turned an Urban Planning System into a Virus Tracking Database," *Technology News*, Reuters, May 22, 2020.

56. "South Korean contact": COVID-19 National Emergency Response Center, Epidemiology & Case Management Team, Korea Centers for Disease Control and Prevention, "Contact Transmission of COVID-19 in South Korea: Novel Investigation Techniques for Tracing Contacts," *Osing Public Health Research Perspective* 11, no. 1 (2020): 60–63. "By obtaining credit": Division of Risk Assessment and International Cooperation, KCDC, "Frequently Asked Questions for KCDC on COVID-19 (Updated on 24 April)."

57. "In South Korea" and "The app also": Government of the Republic of Korea, *Tackling COVID-19 Health, Quarantine and Economic Measures: Korean Experience* (March 31, 2020), 14. "If an exposed": ibid., 13.

58. "To avoid a": "South Korea 'Phone Booth' Coronavirus Tests," *South China Morning Post*, March 19, 2020, https://www.youtube.com/watch?v=A-33i9B8m6E. "Results were available": Government of the Republic of Korea, "Coronavirus-Disease 19: Frequently Asked Questions," http://ncov.mohw.go.kr/en/faqBoardList.do?brdId=13&brdGubun=131&dataGubun=&ncvContSeq=&contSeq=&board_id=&gubun.

59. "Anyone testing positive": Government of Korea, *Tackling COVID-19 Health*, 15. "The government also": Ministry of Public Administration and Security and Ministry of Gender Equality and Family, Government of the Republic of Korea, "To All Koreans Suffering from COVID-19," http://ncov.mohw.go.kr/upload/viewer/skin/doc.html?fn=1589956536786_20200520153536.jpg&rs=/upload/viewer/result/202007/.

60. "But the lessons": Max Fisher and Choe Sang-Hun, "How South Korea Flattened the Curve," *New York Times*, March 23, 2020.

61. "One tool that": COVID-19 National Emergency Response Center et al., "Contact Transmission of COVID-19 in South Korea." "Public health authorities" and "Some districts also": M. S. Kim, "Seoul's Radical Experiment in Digital Contact Tracing," *New Yorker*, April 17, 2020. "COVID-19 is not": Emmanuel Goldman, "Exaggerated Risk of Transmission of COVID-19 by Fomites," *Lancet Infectious Diseases* 20, no. 8, (2020), 892–893, and Kim, "Seoul's Radical Experiment."

62. "In May 2020": Min Joo Kim, "Tracing South Korea's Latest Virus Outbreak Shoves LGBTQ Community into Unwelcome Spotlight," *Washington Post*, May 11, 2020.

Chapter 3

1. "Instead of developing" and "They also need": William Darrow (Professor, Department of Health Promotion and Disease Prevention, Florida International University), interview with the author, June 19, 2020.

2. "This kind of": Mitch Smith et al., "Where Americans Gathered, the Virus Followed," *New York Times*, August 28, 2020.

3. "Cell towers provide": "One of 'High Country' Bandits Sentenced," *Albuquerque Journal*, June 7, 2012, and Phoenix Division, Federal Bureau of Investigation, "'High Country' Bandits Arrested in Arizona," March 12, 2010, accessed July 25, 2020, https://archives.fbi.gov/archives/phoenix/press-releases/2010/px031210.htm. "The CDC suggested": Centers for Disease Control and Prevention, "How Coronavirus Spreads," March 4, 2020. "For asymptomatic carriers": Centers for Disease Control and Prevention, "Coronavirus Disease 2019 (COVID-19): Appendices," May 29, 2020, accessed September 6, 2020, https://www.cdc.gov/coronavirus/2019-ncov/php/contact-tracing/contact-tracing-plan/appendix.html#contact.

4. "The Israeli tool": Tehilla Schwartz Altshuler and Rachel Aridor Herschkowitz, "How Israel's COVID-19 Surveillance Project Works," TechStream, July 6, 2020. "The tool reported": Sergio Perez, "Quarantined after Waving at Coronavirus Patient: How Accurate Is Israel's 'Terrorist-Tracking' Tech?," *Haaretz*, March 18, 2020.

5. Government of the Republic of Korea, "COVID-19, Information Disclosure, such as the Route of Movement of Confirmed Patients (Disease Management Office)," accessed October 26, 2020, https://news.seoul.go.kr/welfare/archives/513105#route_page_top. Once the infectious period is over, detailed information about the infected person's travels is removed from the website.

6. "A smartphone's GPS": gps.gov, "GPS Accuracy," April 22, 2020, accessed July 28. 2020, https://www.gps.gov/systems/gps/performance/accuracy/#commitment.

7. "Even so, GPS": This was the case in Kenya in March 2020; see Cryus Ombati, "State Taps Phones of Isolated Cases," *The Standard*, March 24, 2020. In Ecuador, a presidential decree on March 17, 2020, allowed government authorities to monitor the GPS locations of individuals via their cell phones during the health emergency; see Center for Studies on Freedom

of Expression and Access to Information, "Coronavirus: Data Protection and Confidentiality in Ecuador," and Leon Moreno Garces, *Articulo* 11, no. 1017, March 17, 2020, https://www.defensa.gob.ec/wp-content/uploads /downloads/2020/03/Decreto_presidencial_No_1017_17-Marzo-2020 .pdf. "Throughout the coronavirus": See, e.g., Google, "COVID-19 Community Mobility Reports," accessed July 27, 2020, https://www.google.com /covid19/mobility/. Google's data was anonymized in ways that prevent anyone from gleaning travel information about an individual; see Ahmet Aktay et al., "Google COVID-19 Community Mobility Reports: Anonymization Process Description (Version 1.0)," April 13, 2020, accessed July 27, 2020, https://arxiv.org/pdf/2004.04145.pdf. "In the Netherlands": Jaap van Dissel, chair of the Outbreak Management Team, reported on the Netherlands, accessed July 28, 2020, https://www.youtube.com/watch ?v=OXIIQsjCA98#action=share and Filipino Cabinet Secretary Karlo Nograles reported that Luzon was doing well (https://www.youtube.com /watch?v=k2e9PL8F0dM&t=53m55s). "Washington State drew": Office of the Governor, *Safe Start Washington: A Phased Approach to Recovery*, May 4, 2020, 2.

8. "TraceFi was based": In order for this to actually work, Harvard increased the number of Wi-Fi receptors though the use of Raspberry Pis, cheap, single-board computers. This has been done in a limited number of buildings (Jim Waldo, Gordon McKay Professor of the Practice of Computer Science, Harvard University, interview with the author, September 3, 2020). "Such information can": "TraceFi," Harvard University, accessed September 3, 2020, https://covidtech.harvard.edu/howitworks.html.

9. "When users sign": Originally, only a phone number was needed for registration; the requirement for using identity verification occurred in Version 2.0 of the app in August 2020 (Ministry of Health, Government of Singapore, "App Release Notes, Version 2.0," https://support.tracetogether .gov.sg/hc/en-sg/articles/360046481013-App-Release-Notes). "This is a": Ministry of Health, Government of Singapore, "Launch of New App for Contact Tracing," accessed July 28, 2020, https://www.smartnation.gov .sg/docs/default-source/press-release-materials/sndgg_tracetogether ---media-factsheet.pdf?sfvrsn=8e956b90_2. "To protect users": The open source version recommends changing identifiers every fifteen minutes (see Jason Bay et al., "BlueTrace: A Privacy-Preserving Protocol for Community-Driven Contact Tracing across Borders," accessed July 29,

2020, https://bluetrace.io/static/bluetrace_whitepaper-938063656596c104 632def383eb33b3c.pdf, 2); there is no official documentation on how frequently the TraceTogether identifiers are changed. "An MOH server": Ministry of Health, Government of Singapore, "Launch of New App for Contact Tracing," and Team TraceTogether, Government of Singapore, "App Release Notes," accessed August 13, 2020, Version 1.6, https://support .tracetogether.gov.sg/hc/en-sg/articles/360046481013-App-Release-Notes.

10. "If Ben were": Bay, "BlueTrace," 4. "If so, MOH": Team TraceTogether, Government of Singapore, "TraceTogether Privacy Safeguards," accessed September 1, 2020, https://www.tracetogether.gov.sg/common/privacystate ment. "The health ministry": Team TraceTogether, Government of Singapore, "Can I Say No to Uploading my TraceTogether Data When Contacted by the Ministry of Health?," accessed July 28, 2020, https://support .tracetogether.gov.sg/hc/en-sg/articles/360044860414-Can-I-say-no-to -uploading-my-TraceTogether-data-when-contacted-by-the-Ministry-of -Health-.

11. "Because Alyssa was": MOH supplies the temporary identifiers to the users, so it can link users to these temporary identifiers. "Contacting everyone associated": Bay, "BlueTrace," 5.

12. "Ben's singing with": Lea Hammer et al., "High SARS-CoV-2 Attack Rate Following Exposure at a Choir Practice—Skagit County, Washington, March 2020," *Morbidity and Mortality Weekly Report* 69, no. 19 (May 15, 2020): 606–610. "Then, and only": Bay, "BlueTrace," 4–5, 6. "MOH also obtains": Ministry of Health, Government of Singapore, "Launch of New App for Contact Tracing."

13. "Apple's iPhones use" and "Health authorities in": Bay, "BlueTrace," 7. "Later the TraceTogether": Team TraceTogether, Government of Singapore, "I see 'COVID-19 Exposure Notifications' in my phone's operating system. Do I need to turn it on for my TraceTogether app to work in the background?," accessed August 31, 2020, https://support.tracetogether .gov.sg/hc/en-sg/articles/360050556334-I-see-COVID-19-Exposure-Notifi cations-in-my-phone-s-operating-system-Do-I-need-to-turn-it-on-for -my-TraceTogether-app-to-work-in-the-background-.

14. "In April 2020": Jesse Yeung and Isaac Yee, "Tens of Thousands of Singapore Migrant Workers Are Infected. The Rest Are Stuck in Their Dorms as the Country Opens Up," CNN, May 14, 2020. "The outbreak

occurred": Shabani Mahtani, "Singapore Lost Control of Its Coronavirus Outbreak, and Migrant Workers Are the Victims," *Washington Post*, April 21, 2020, accessed July 29, 2020, https://www.cnn.com/2020/05/14/asia /singapore-migrant-worker-coronavirus-intl-hnk/index.html. "The Singaporean government": Ministry of Manpower, Government of Singapore, "FAQs on Using TraceTogether," *BBC News*, July 1, 2020, accessed July 28, 2020, https://www.mom.gov.sg/covid-19/frequently-asked-questions /tracetogether.

15. "A study from" and "Singapore's experience shows": Robert Hinch et al., "Effective Configurations of a Digital Contact Tracing App: A Report to NHSX," technical report, NHSX, April 2020, https://cdn.theconversation .com/staticfiles/files/1009/Report-EffectiveAppConfigurations.pdf?1587 531217. "Singapore's experience shows": Saira Asher, "Coronavirus: Why Singapore Turned to Wearable Contact-Tracing Tech," *BBC News*, July 5, 2020.

16. "If someone tested": "Improving TraceTogether through Community Engagement," GovTech Singapore, July 6, 2020, accessed September 1, 2020, https://www.tech.gov.sg/media/technews/2020-07-06-tracetogether -token-teardown. "The first distribution": "Coronavirus: 10,000 seniors get first batch of TraceTogether tokens," StraitTimes, July 7, 2020.

17. "Anyone entering a": Government of Singapore, "SafeEntry FAQ," accessed August 24, 2020, https://covid.gobusiness.gov.sg/faq/safeentry, and Government of Singapore, "SafeEntry: What's New," https://www .safeentry.gov.sg/latest_news#news-15, May 27, 2020.

18. "Schools required students": "Linking Midday Meal to Aadhaar Is Wrong," *Deccan Herald*, March 11, 2017, accessed August 13, 2020, http:// www.deccanherald.com/content/600599/linking-midday-meal-aadhaar -wrong.html, and Sanyatan Bera, "Why Aadhaar Is Mandatory for Temple Rituals at Tirupati," *LiveMint*, July 26, 2016. "Aadhaar's introduction was": Pam A. Dixon, "A Failure to 'Do No Harm'—India's Aadhaar Biometric ID Program and Its Inability to Protect Privacy in Relation to Measures in Europe and the U.S.," *Technology Science* 7 (2017), 539–567. As Dixon noted, the program lacked fundamental privacy protections, from the ability of a citizen to opt out (obtaining government benefits becomes essentially impossible without an Aadhaar ID) to obtaining proper redress when privacy violations occurred.

19. "When users register": Government of India, "Privacy Policy," 1, accessed August 8, 2020, https://static.mygov.in/rest/s3fs-public/mygov_15905164 5651307401.pdf. "Aarogya Setu then": "Aarogya Setu App: Follow the Simple Steps to Do a Self-Assessment Test," *India Today*, May 2, 2020, accessed September 1, 2020, https://www.indiatoday.in/information/story /aarogya-setu-app-follow-these-simple-steps-to-do-a-self-assessment-test -1673656-2020-05-02.

20. "The app provides": Ashok Jhunjhunwala, "Role of Telecom Network to Manage COVID-19 in India: Aarogya Setu," *Transactions of the Indian National Academy of Engineering*, 2020, 1–5, advance online publication, https://doi.org/10.1007/s41403-020-00109-7. "In many places": Arunabh Saikia, "Covid-19: As Cases Surge across India, Many States Abandon Contact Tracing," *Scroll.in*, July 13, 2020, and Jeremy Gittleman and Sameer Yasir, "India's Covid Outbreak Is Now the World's Fastest Growing," *New York Times*, August 28, 2020.

21. "In a podcast": Lalitesh Katragadda, "Aarogya Setu: A Surveillance App?," in "Interview: Is Aarogya Setu a Tool for Covid-19 Contact Tracing or Mass Surveillance?," *Scroll.in*, April 20, 2020, 6:42–6:48. "Within weeks of": Ministry of Electronics and Information Technology, Electronic Niketan, CGO Complex, New Delhi, "Aarogya Setu Is Now Open Source," May 26, 2020, accessed August 8, 2020, https://static.mygov.in/rest/s3fs -public/mygov_159050700051307401.pdf. "Raman Jit Singh": Raman Jit Singh Chima (Senior International Counsel and Asia Pacific Policy Direc- tor), interview with the author, September 4, 2020. "He added later": Chima, personal communication, September 8, 2020.

22. "This function works": Lalitesh Katragadda (Lead Volunteer, Head of Product and Architecture, Aarogya Setu), personal communication, August 26, 2020.

23. "In contrast to": The static IDs are called unique IDs; see Government of India, "Aarogya Setu Privacy Policy," 1 a and b, accessed August 26, 2020, https://static.mygov.in/rest/s3fs-public/mygov_159051645651307401.pdf. "The Indian Army": Amrita Nayak Dutta, "Army Advises Personnel to Use Aarogya Setu App, but with Usual Cybersecurity Precautions," *ThePrint*, April 15, 2020.

24. "But if Bharghav": Government of India, "Aarogya Setu Privacy Policy," 2, accessed August 22, 2020, https://static.mygov.in/rest/s3fs-publicmygov

_159051645651307401.pdf. There is no date on the document, but various newspaper articles date this from mid- to late May 2020; see, e.g., Aditi Agrawal, "Aarogya Setu Updates Privacy Policy, Terms of Service: Reverse Engineering not Banned, but Function Creep Now Legitimized," *Medianama*, May 24, 2020, https://perma.cc/89JY-6GKE.

25. "In early May": Ministry of Home Affairs, Government of India, Order, No. 40-3/2020-DM-I(A), May 1, 2020, 2 and 7, accessed August 21, 2020, https:/perma.cc/6SW7-779. "That order was": K. J. Shashidhar, "Aarogya Setu and Its Many Conflicts," Observer Research Foundation, June 6, 2020, accessed August 8, 2020, https://www.orfonline.org/expert-speak /aarogya-setu-app-many-conflicts-67442/. "Some shopping malls": Aditi Agrawal, "Dehli Mall Requires Aarogya Setu to Visit Grocery Store, PIL Filed in Dehli HC," *Medianama*, May 22, 2020; Team Herald, "Chaos at S Goa Collectorate after Public Denied Entry sans Aarogya Setu App's 'Safe' Message," *Herald*, July 22, 2020; and "Denied Medicine for Parents Claims Noida Man as Society Seeks Aarogya Setu," *Indian Express*, April 24, 2020. "Several months later": "Aarogya Setu's New Feature to Help Organisations Get Health Status of Staff, Other Users," *Economic Times*, August 22, 2020.

26. "When it comes": McKinsey Global Institute, "Digital India: Technology to Transform a Connected Nation," March 2019, 34.

27. "An Aadhaar number": National Institute for Transforming India, Government of India, "National Health Stack: Strategy and Approach," July 2018, 28. "It's notable that": ibid., 27.

28. "Katragadda said that": Priyali Sur, "Many Indian Citizens Believe Their Government Is Trying to Steal and Sell Their Data. Here's Why," *CNN Business*, June 21, 2020. "He assured me": Lalitesh Katragadda (Lead Volunteer, Head of Product and Architecture, Aarogya Setu), personal communication, September 3, 2020. "That claim, however": Government of India, Ministry of Electronics and Information Technology, "Order. Subject: Notification of the Aarogya Setu Data Access and Knowledge Sharing Protocol, 2020 in Light of the COVID-19 Pandemic," May 11, 2020, accessed September 2, 2020, https://www.meity.gov.in/writereaddata/files /Aarogya_Setu_data_access_knowledge_Protocol.pdf. "But an analysis": Internet Freedom Foundation, "Summary and Analysis of the Aarogya Setu Data Access and Knowledge Sharing Protocol, 2020," May 13, 2020, accessed September 6, 2020, https://drive.google.com/file/d/1CsDRlM

DvqAH1Dq2xU5nP7GxdnDPIKhWp/view. "Of greatest concern": Government of India, Ministry of Electronics and Information Technology, "Order. Subject: Notification of the Aarogya Setu Data Access and Knowledge Sharing Protocol," "Implementation of the Protocol," 5d, "Rationale for This Protocol," 2 and 3. "IFF also noted": Internet Freedom Foundation, "Summary and Analysis of the Aarogya Setu Data Access and Knowledge Sharing Protocol, 2020," 28C and 28D.

29. "Without even a": Altshuler and Herschkowitz, "How Israel's COVID-19." "The country used": Joe Tidy, "Coronavirus: Israel Enables Emergency Spy Powers," BBC, March 17, 2020, https://www.bbc.com/news/technology-51930681.

Chapter 4

1. "During the height": AP, "14-Year-Old with AIDS Attends School after Two Years," *New York Times*, August 26, 1986; William Grady, Bill Crawford, and John O'Brien, "Baker and MacKenzie Fined in AIDS Case," *Chicago Tribune*, January 11, 1994; and "When Doctors Refuse to Treat AIDS," *New York Times*, August 3, 1987.

2. "A trip to": Douglas Ginsburg, *U.S. v. Maynard*, 615 F. 3rd 544 (D.C. Circuit 2010), 29–30.

3. "It's easy to": Yves-Alexandre de Montjoye, Cesar A. Hidalgo, Michel Verleysen, and Vincent D. Blondel, "Unique in the Crowd: The Privacy Bounds of Human Mobility," *Scientific Reports* 3 (2013). Of course, this information is less useful if people are only at home while obeying "stay safe, stay home" orders.

4. "Your social network": M. Keith Chen and Ryne Rohla, "The Effect of Partisanship and Political Advertising on Close Family Ties," *Science* 360, no. 6392 (June 1, 2018): 1020–1024; Carter Jernigan and Bertram T. Mistree, "Gaydar: Facebook Friendships Expose Sexual Orientation," *First Monday* 14, no. 10 (2009).

5. "'I was not'": Carmela Troncoso (Professor, Security and Privacy Engineering Lab, École Polytechnique Féderalé Lausanne), interview with the author, August 4, 2020. "With infections soaring": Apoorva Mandavilli, "First Documented Coronavirus Reinfection Reported in Hong Kong,"

New York Times, August 24, 2020. "Looking at the": Troncoso, interview with the author, August 4, 2020.

6. "Three groups of": Decentralized Privacy-Preserving Proximity Tracing (DP3T), and two from the U.S. named PACT, later distinguished as PACT-E and PACT-W—for East and West Coasts, independently hit upon the same technical scheme, which they rapidly went about implementing. PACT-E's name comes from Private Automated Contact Tracing, while PACT-W's is from their paper: "PACT: Privacy Sensitive Protocols and Mechanisms for Mobile Contact Tracing." PACT-W is now known as Common Circle. "Meanwhile Google and": Apple makes its phones. Google develops the Android software, but the phones are made by various manufacturers. Together the Android and iOS operating systems are used by 95.5 percent of the world's mobile devices (Mobile Operating Market Share Worldwide, https://gs.statcounter.com/os-market-share/mobile/worldwide). The method for using the phones for notifications is described in Apple, "Privacy-Preserving Contact Tracing," accessed August 6, 2020, https://www.apple.com/covid19/contacttracing. "The app would": This statement is not absolute. There are various ways that a person could determine who exposed them. For example, if someone publicly released information about Bobby's testing positively for COVID-19, or if Aliyah only rarely leaves her apartment, she may be able to determine when she was exposed to COVID-19, and who exposed her.

7. "This preserves the": Android phones also had a battery drain problem when doing continuous BLE scanning that was resolved similarly.

8. "The companies agreed": Google, "Google COVID-19 Exposure Notifications Service Additional Terms," May 4, 2020, accessed September 5, 2020, https://blog.google/documents/72/Exposure_Notifications_Service_Additional_Terms.pdf.

9. "No one learns": Of course, Aliyah may figure this out from other information, including Bobby telling her. The point is that the app does not release the information.

10. "'Suppose you are'": Richard Rothenberg (Regents Professor, Georgia State University School of Public Health), interview with the author, June 17, 2020.

11. "Sometimes people think" and "She explained, 'Whereas'": Kate Adern, "The Trouble with England's Test-and-Trace System," *Guardian*, August

20, 2020, 14:58–15:37, https://www.theguardian.com/news/audio/2020/aug/20/the-trouble-with-englands-test-and-trace-system-podcast.

12. "Bart's phone then": The situation is actually somewhat more complex than described in the text. The GAEN system uses a Temporary Exposure Key (TEK) that changes daily and that is calculated by the phone itself. Each day the phone computes the rolling proximity identifiers (RPIs) from the TEK. If Bart tests positive and enters a valid verification code, his phone uploads the TEKs it used during the period when he was infectious to the health authority's server. From this information, the health authority can calculate the RPIs that Bart's phone broadcast during his infectious period. The reason for sending the health authority ten days' worth of TEKs, rather than the used RPIs, is that transmitting the former consumes much less bandwidth than the thousand RPIs used over the period.

13. "There's some variability": This statement was accurate as of August 2020. If an app is running on background on an iPhone, then it samples every two and a half minutes.

14. "At that point": For privacy reasons, GAEN limits an app to six queries every twenty-four hours (this is for version 1.5 of the GAEN infrastructure). This prevents an app from pinpointing the moment when someone's identifiers are added to the system—and thus figuring out when exposure happened and thus perhaps who it was.

15. "Amelie's app then": Of course, it could be that Alyssa was on the bus with Daryll and Emilia at 7:30 am and wasn't near Bart until lunchtime. If the app is checking in at 8 am, the 7:30 am exposure would be included in the previous day's cumulative exposure, and SwissCovid will not warn Alyssa of her risk. That's why Alyssa's phone does a second check with the health authority at 8 pm. When SwissCovid queries the identifiers from the previous twenty-four hours, Daryll and Emilia's exposure will now be in the same "slice" of day as Bart's; Alyssa will receive a notification that she was exposed. "If yes, Amelie": Federal Office of Public Health, Switzerland, "New Coronavirus: Frequently Asked Questions (FAQ)," August 3, 2020, https://www.bag.admin.ch/bag/en/home/krankheiten/ausbrueche-epidemien-pandemien/aktuelle-ausbrueche-epidemien/novel-cov/faq-kontakte-downloads/haeufig-gestellte-fragen.html?faq-url=/en/swisscovid-app-coronavirus-test-positive/what-should-i-do-if-swisscovid-app-alerts-me-about-0. "She's also told": Federal Office of Public Health,

Switzerland, "New Coronavirus: Frequently Asked Questions (FAQ)," August 3, 2020, https://www.bag.admin.ch/bag/en/home/krankheiten/aus brueche-epidemien-pandemien/aktuelle-ausbrueche-epidemien/novel-cov /faq-kontakte-downloads/haeufig-gestellte-fragen.html?faq-url=/en/swiss covid-app-examples-cases/i-have-received-alert-swisscovid-app-saying -possibility-infection-4.

16. "The Swiss government": Le conseil federale, Government of Switzerland, "Allocation pour perte de gain en cas de mesures destinées à lutter contre le coronavirus," accessed August 11, 2020, https://www.bsv.admin .ch/bsv/fr/home/sozialversicherungen/eo-msv/grundlagen-und-gesetze /eo-corona.html.

17. "The survey starts" and "If a user": Government of the Republic of Ireland, HSE, "How the COVID Tracker App Works," accessed August 27, 2020, https://covidtracker.gov.ie/how-the-app-works/.

18. "If a COVID": Government of the Republic of Ireland, HSE, "Privacy and How We Use Your Data," accessed August 27, 2020, https://covidtracker .gov.ie/privacy-and-data/. "Otherwise, Aoife will": Government of Ireland, "How COVID Tracker App Works." "In either case": Colm Harte (Technical Director, Nearform), personal communication, September 4, 2020.

19. "The app appears": Charlotte Jee, "Is a Successful Contact-Tracing App Possible? These Countries Think So," *MIT Technology Review*, August 10, 2020.

20. "With the user's" and "Ireland's Health Services": Government of the Republic of Ireland, HSE, "Data Protection Information Notice Covid Tracker App," 5.4: What App Metrics Are Collected, accessed September 5, 2020, https://covidtracker.gov.ie/privacy-and-data/data-protection/#5.4.

21. "The national organization": Association of Public Health Laboratories, "Bringing COVID-19 Exposure Notification to the Public Health Community," July 17, 2020, accessed August 24, 2020, https://www.aphl blog.org/bringing-covid-19-exposure-notification-to-the-public-health -community/.

22. "To qualify, apps": European Commission, "Coronavirus: A Common Approach for Safe and Efficient Mobile Tracing Apps across the EU," May 13, 2020, accessed September 9, 2020, https://ec.europa.eu/commission /presscorner/detail/en/qanda_20_869.

23. "Privacy was the": Carmela Troncoso, interview with the author, August 4, 2020.

24. "And while many": Daniel J. Solove, "'I've Got Nothing to Hide' and Other Misunderstandings of Privacy," *San Diego Law Review* 44 (2007): 749.

25. This discussion is based in part on Vanessa Teague, "Contact Tracing without Surveillance," April 7, 2020, accessed August 26, 2020, https:// github.com/vteague/contactTracing/blob/master/blog/2020-04-07Contact TracingWithoutSurveillance.md.

26. "Or they might": Northeastern University expelled eleven students for violating rules about large gatherings; apps were not involved in the discovery of this gathering. See Ian Thomsen, "Northeastern Dismisses 11 Students for Gathering in Violation of COVID-19 Policies," *News@Northeastern*, September 4, 2020.

27. "This enables organizations": Internet Freedom Foundation, "We Studied the Protocol: And No, This Doesn't Sufficiently Protect Your Privacy," May 13, 2020, accessed September 5, 2020, https://internetfreedom.in /we-studied-the-protocol-and-no-this-doesnt-sufficiently-protect-your -privacy/. *MIT Technology Review* has been tracking apps from around the world and rating how well they do in terms of different aspects of privacy (see Patrick Howell O'Neill, Tate Ryan-Mosley, and Bobbie Johnson, "A Flood of Coronavirus Apps Are Tracking Us. Now It's Time to Keep Track of Them," *MIT Technology Review*, May 7, 2020).

28. "The two GAEN": Kobi Leins, Christopher Culnane, and Ben I. P. Rubenstein, "Tracking, Tracing, Trust: Contemplating Mitigating the Impact of COVID-19 through Technological Interventions," *Medical Journal of Australia* 213, no. 1 (2020). "But while Aarogya": The app code is public, but the underlying computations on the server are not; see Jagmeet Singh, "Aarogya Setu iOS Version Gets Open Sourced over Two Months after Promise," *Gadgets360*, August 13, 2020.

29. "Adversaries can come": George Ellard, Inspector General, NSA, Letter to Senator Charles Grassley, September 13, 2013, accessed September 10, 2020, https://www.nsa.gov/Portals/70/documents/news-features/press -room/statements/grassley-letter.pdf. "GAEN-based and": Carmela Troncoso et al., "Decentralized Privacy-Preserving Proximity Tracking," 22–25,

May 25, 2020, https://github.com/DP-3T/documents/blob/master/DP3T%20White%20Paper.pdf.

30. "But like any": One such possibility is the so-called replay attack, in which an adversary collects temporary IDs near a hospital, then "replays" them at a location with lots of people (e.g., a train station). The phones there pick up the temporary IDs, some of which are likely to later be reported as belonging to someone who is infected with COVID-19. See, e.g., Schewiezerische Eidgenossenschaft, Eidgenössisches Finanzdepartemente, "Replay Attacks," 2, June 14, 2020, https://www.melani.admin.ch/dam/melani/de/dokumente/2020/Replay-Attacks-Risk-Estimation_Public_Signed.pdf.download.pdf/Replay-Attacks-Risk-Estimation_Public_Signed.pdf.

Chapter 5

1. "It continued to": "New York," accessed September 4, 2020, https://rt.live/us/NY.

2. "Participants agreed to": Petra Klepac, Stephen Kissler, and Julia Gog, "Contagion! The BBC Four Pandemic: The Model behind the Documentary," *Epidemics* 24 (2018): 49–59.

3. "The data allowed": Petra Klepac, Adam J. Kucharski, Andrew J. K. Conlan, et al., "Contacts in Context: Large-Scale Setting-Specific Social Mixing Matrices from the BBC Pandemic Project," Version 2.0, March 2020, https://www.medrxiv.org/content/medrxiv/early/2020/03/05/2020.02.16.20023754.full.pdf, and Adam J. Kucharski et al., "Effectiveness of Isolation, Testing, Contact Tracing, and Physical Distancing on Reducing Transmission of SARS-CoV-2 in Different Settings: A Mathematical Modelling Study," *Lancet Infectious Diseases*, June 16, 2020, https://doi.org/10.1016/S1473-2099(20)30457-6.

4. "The resulting model," "If 90 percent," "In another iteration," and "By notifying people": Kucharski et al., "Effectiveness of Isolation."

5. "The claims that": The paper assumes that all who install the app will also use them (Adam Kucharski, Associate Professor and Sir Henry Dale Fellow, Department of Epidemiology at the London School of Hygiene and Tropical Medicine, personal communication, October 27, 2020). Full use of the app after installation is highly unlikely.

6. "If the apps": Susan Landau, "Location Surveillance to Counter COVID-19: Efficacy Is What Matters," *Lawfare*, March 25, 2020.

7. "For the CDC": Centers for Disease Control and Prevention, "How to Protect Yourself & Others," July 31, 2020, https://www.cdc.gov/coronavirus /2019-ncov/prevent-getting-sick/prevention.html.

8. "To test the": Steffen Meyer et al., "Google Exposure Notification API," accessed August 17, 2020, https://github.com/corona-warn-app/cwa-docu mentation/blob/master/2020_06_24_Corona_API_measurements.pdf, and Fraunhofer, "Press Release: Key Contribution to Containing the Coronavirus Pandemic, Fraunhofer Assists with the Development of the Coronavirus Warning App," June 16, 2020. "Over 139 tests": Meyer et al., "Google Exposure Notification API," 21. "The 'train car'": ibid., 5, 8, 11, and 18.

9. "When researchers from": Douglas Leith and Stephen J. Farrell, "Measurement-Based Evaluation of Google/Apple Exposure Notification API for Proximity Detection in a Light-Rail Tram," *PLoS One* 5, no. 9 (September 2020). "Seven volunteers with": The Dublin testers used Google Pixel 2s, while the Fraunhofer experimenters used Google Pixel 4s; this distinction should not matter. See Leith and Farrell, "Measurement-Based Evaluation." "Apparently a flexible": ibid.

10. "The signal strength": Douglas J. Leith and Stephen Farrell, "Coronavirus Contact Tracing: Evaluating the Potential of Using Bluetooth Received Signal Strength for Proximity Detection," May 6, 2020, 4, https://www.scss .tcd.ie/Doug.Leith/pubs/bluetooth_rssi_study.pdf.

11. "When an infected" and "The smallest of": Mahesh Jayaweera et al., "Transmission of COVID-19 Virus by Droplets and Aerosols: A Critical Review on the Unresolved Dichotomy," *Environmental Research* 188 (September 2020): 109819, https://doi.org/10.1016/j.envres.2020.109819. "The bigger ones": Jasmin S. Kutter et al., "Transmission Routes of Respiratory Viruses among Humans," *Current Opinion in Virology* 28 (2018): 142–151, https://doi.org/10.1016/j.coviro.2018.01.001. "This is apparently" and "One was at": Liu et al., "COVID-19 Outbreak Associated with Air Conditioning in Restaurant, Guangzhou, China," *Emerging Infectious Diseases* 26, no. 7 (July 2020).

12. "A review of": This is based on a review of a number of cases; see Daniel P. Oran and Eric J. Topol, "Prevalence of Asymptomatic SARS-CoV-2 Infection: A Narrative Review," *Annals of Internal Medicine* (2020), https://

doi.org/10.7326/M20-3012. "While these studies": D. F. Gudbjartsson et al., "Spread of SARS-CoV-2 in the Icelandic Population," *New England Journal of Medicine* 382, no. 24 (June 11, 2020): 3214. "Even if one": Seyed Moghadas et al., "The Implications of Silent Transmission for the Control of COVID-19 Outbreaks," *Proceedings of the National Academies of Science* 117, no. 30 (2020).

13. "Virginia's website for": Virginia Department of Health, "COVIDWISE Frequently Asked Questions," accessed September 5, 2020, https://www.vdh.virginia.gov/covidwise/frequently-asked-questions/. "When tested in": Mark Briers, "A Technical Roadmap for the U.K.'s Contact Tracing Functionality: A Successful App Is Appropriately Able to Assess Risk," Alan Turing Institute blog, August 13, 2020, https://www.turing.ac.uk/blog/technical-roadmap-uks-contract-tracing-app-functionality. "These numbers sound": Mark Briers (Professor and Programme Director for Defence and Security and Co-Chair of the Research and Innovation Advisory Committee, Turing Institute, University of Cambridge), interview with the author, September 17, 2020.

14. "For these workers" and "What's more, many": Susan Landau, Christy Lopez, and Laura Moy, "The Importance of Equity in Contact Tracing," *Lawfare*, May 1, 2020, https://www.lawfareblog.com/importance-equity-contact-tracing. "Similarly, people who": Douglas J. Leith and Stephen Farrell, "Coronavirus Contact Tracing: Evaluating the Potential of Using Bluetooth Received Signal Strength for Proximity Detection," May 6, 2020, 5, https://www.scss.tcd.ie/Doug.Leith/pubs/bluetooth_rssi_study.pdf.

15. "The city has": As of September 9, 2020, Chelsea had had 3,448 infections in an estimated population of 40,000 people; the state had 121,396 cases in an estimated population of 6.893 million, while Boston had 16,568 positives in an estimated population of 695,000 (Massachusetts Department of Public Health, "COVID-19 Dashboard—Wednesday, September 09, 2020, Weekly COVID-19 Public Health Report," accessed September 12, 2020, https://www.mass.gov/doc/weekly-covid-19-public-health-report-september-9-2020/download).

16. "Chelsea's population is": The city is two-thirds Latinx (Jose A. Del Real, "In an Immigrant Community Battling Coronavirus, 'Essential' Means 'Vulnerable,'" *Washington Post*, May 9, 2020). The infection rate is from Centers for Disease Control and Prevention, "COVID-19 Hospitalization and Death by Race/Ethnicity," August 18, 2020, https://www

.cdc.gov/coronavirus/2019-ncov/covid-data/investigations-discovery /hospitalization-death-by-race-ethnicity.html. "Almost half are": Jose Figueroa, "Harvard Researcher Discusses Why COVID-19 Is Devastating Communities of Color," NPR Health Watch, September 6, 2020, https:// www.npr.org/2020/09/06/910194836/harvard-researcher-discusses-why -covid-19-is-devastating-communities-of-color, and Jose Figueroa et al., "Community-Level Factors Associated with Racial and Ethnic Disparities in COVID-19 Rates in Massachusetts," *Health Affairs* 39, no. 11 (November 2020). "Looking at COVID": ibid. and Elizabeth Cooney, "Immigration Status, Housing, and Food-Service Work Explain Covid-19's Burden on Latinos," *Stat*, August 27, 2020, accessed September 30, 2020, https:// www.statnews.com/2020/08/27/three-factors-explain-covid19-burden -on-latinos/.

17. "In February 2020" and "One consequence is": Benjamin Sommers et al., "Assessment of Perceptions of the Public Charge Rule among Low-Income Adults in Texas," *JAMA Network Open* 3, no. 7 (2020).

18. "In Chelsea, few" and "Alexander Train, assistant": Ellen Barry, "In a Crowded City, Leaders Struggle to Separate the Sick from the Well," *New York Times*, April 25, 2020.

19. "Twenty-three percent": Elliot Ramos and María Inés Zamiudo, "In Chicago, 70% of COVID-19 Deaths Are Black," WBEZ, April 5, 2020. "By then, it": As of mid-August 2020, per 100,000 people, Black Americans have experienced a death rate of 88.4; the indigenous community, 73.2; Latinx, 54.4; and white Americans, 40.4 (APM Research Lab Staff, "The Color of Coronavirus: COVID-19 Deaths by Race and Ethnicity in the U.S.," August 19, 2020, https://www.apmresearchlab.org/covid/deaths-by-race).

20. "Black Americans are": Figueroa et al., "Community-Level Factors"; Josefa Velasquez et al., "COVID Sends Public Housing-Zone Residents to Hospitals at Unusually High Rates," *The City*, May 14, 2020; Gregorio A. Millett et al., "Assessing Differential Impacts of COVID-19 on Black Communities," *Annals of Epidemiology* 47 (July 2020): 37044; and Monica Anderson, "Who Relies on Public Transit in the U.S.," Pew Research Center, April 7, 2016. "Decades of federal": U.S. Commission on Civil Rights, *Understanding Fair Housing*, Clearinghouse Publication 42 (February 1973): 3–5, and Terry Gross, "A 'Forgotten History' of How the U.S. Government Segregated America," Fresh Air, May 3, 2017, https:// www.npr.org/2017/05/03/526655831/a-forgotten-history-of-how-the-u

-s-government-segregated-america. "Discriminatory housing policies": Linda Villarosa, "Pollution Is Killing Black Americans. This Community Fought Back," *New York Times Magazine*, July 28, 2020. "Adding to this": Kelly M. Bower et al., "The Intersection of Neighborhood Racial Segregation, Poverty, and Urbanicity and Its Impact on Food Store Availability in the United States," *Preventive Medicine* 58 (2014): 33–39, https://doi.org/10.1016/j.ypmed.2013.10.010.

21. "The result is": APM Research Lab, "The Color of Coronavirus: COVID-19 Deaths by Race and Ethnicity in the U.S.," October 15, 2020, accessed October 20, 2020, https://www.apmresearchlab.org/covid/deaths-by-race.

22. "Centuries of racism": John Eligon and Audra D. S. Burch, "Questions of Bias in Covid-19 Treatment Add to the Mourning in Black Families," *New York Times*, May 10, 2020. "Others including denying": Elizabeth Grennan Browning, "Those Most at Risk Might Be Most Wary of a Coronavirus Vaccine," *Washington Post*, September 11, 2020; Rebecca Skloot, *The Immortal Life of Henrietta Lacks* (New York: Crown, 2010); and Maya Overby Koretzky, "'A Change of Heart': Racial Politics, Scientific Metaphor and Coverage of 1968 Interracial Heart Transplants in the African American Press," *Social History of Medicine: the Journal of the Society for the Social History of Medicine* 30, no. 2 (2017): 408–428, https://doi.org/10.1093/shm/hkw052. "A 2002 Institute" and "Black American were": Institute of Medicine, *Unequal Treatment: Confronting Racial and Ethnic Disparities in Health Care* (Washington, DC: National Academies Press, 2002), https://doi.org/10.17226/12875. "Such disparities in": ibid. and "Long-Standing Racial and Income Disparities Seen Creeping into COVID-19 Care," KHN, April 6, 2020, accessed October 1, 2020, https://khn.org/news/covid-19-treatment-racial-income-health-disparities/.

23. "Howard Brown Health," "Contact tracers began," and "They provided infected": John A. Schneider and Harold A. Pollack, "Flipping the Script for Coronavirus Disease 2019 Contact Tracing," *JAMA Network*, September 16, 2020.

24. "John Hopkins University's": Emily Gurley, "Balancing Public Good with Privacy, Autonomy, and Confidentiality," COVID-19 Contact Tracing, Coursera, 6:40–7:44.

25. "Some members of": Lauren Bavis, "Advocates Worry Contact Tracing Leaves Black, Latinx Communities Behind," Indiana Public Media,

September 18, 2020, https://indianapublicmedia.org/news/advocates-worry
-contact-tracing-leaves-black,-latinx-communities-behind.php.

26. "Zinzi Bailey, a," "'In a neighborhood,'" and "Baily explained, 'An'":
Zinzi Bailey (Assistant Scientist, University of Miami Miller School of
Medicine), interview with the author, June 18, 2020.

27. "Despite a chronic": Mark Walker, "Pandemic Highlights Deep-Rooted
Problems in Indian Health Service," *New York Times*, September 29, 2020,
and Ryan M. Close and Myles J. Stone, "Contact Tracing for Native Americans in Rural Arizona," *New England Journal of Medicine* 383 (2020). "It
relied heavily": ibid.

28. "Children in Apache": Kathleen Bahr, "The Strengths of Apache Grandmothers: Observations on Commitment, Culture, and Caretaking," *Journal
of Comparative Family Studies* 25, no. 2 (Summer 1994): 233–248. "Instead
of asking": Close and Stone, "Contact Tracing for Native Americans." "If
someone was": Allee Mead, "Contact Tracing: Training New Workers and
Connecting with Rural Residents," *The Rural Monitor*, September 9, 2020.

29. "Then, suddenly, they're" and "With COVID, early": Jennifer Couzin-
Frankel, "The Mystery of the Pandemic's 'Happy Hypoxia,'" *Science* 368, no.
4690 (2020): 455–456.

30. "When the Disease": Mead, "Contact Tracing."

31. "Despite the reservation's": Gina Kolata, "On Native American Land,
Contact Tracing is Saving Lives," *New York Times,* August 13, 2020. "The
intervention was": Close and Stone, "Contact Tracing for Native Americans." "The medical teams": Mead, "Contact Tracing."

32. "In Germany, testing": Tamara Kovacevic and Ben Butcher, "Covid
in Europe: How Much Testing Do Other Countries Do?," *BBC News*, September 19, 2020, https://www.bbc.com/news/54181291. "France has been":
Aurelian Breeden, "France to Smooth Snarled Testing Process as Virus Pressure Grows," *New York Times*, September 11, 2020. "In the UK": Gareth Iaco-
bucci, "Covid-19: Testing Service Wasn't Prepared for Increased Demand,
Chief Admits," *British Medical Journal* 370 (September 18, 2020). "Backlogs
are anticipated": *BBC News*, "Not Enough Tests due to Winter Coughs," September 16, 2020, https://www.bbc.com/news/health-54175451. "In October
2020": Keith Collins, "Is Your State Doing Enough Coronavirus Testing?,"
New York Times, October 2, 2020.

33. "The *Wall Street*": Matthew Dalton, "Contact Tracing, the West's Big Hope for Suppressing Covid-19, Is in Disarray," *Wall Street Journal*, September 17, 2020. "Annoyed about spam": Bryan Pietsch, "Coronavirus Tracers Beg Residents: Please Answer Your Phones," *New York Times*, September 29, 2020. "New York State": Jennifer Peltz, "'Are You Doing OK': On the Ground with NYC Contact Tracers," NBCNewYork, August 17, 2020, https://www.nbcnewyork.com/news/local/are-you-doing-ok-on-the-ground-with-nyc-contact-tracers/2570393. "In Maryland and": ibid.; Elliot Williams, Jenny Gathright, and Daniella Cheslow, "As Contact Tracing Ramps Up in the D.C. Region, What Have We Learned So Far?," WAMU, August 11, 2020, https://wamu.org/story/20/08/11/dc-md-va-region-contact-tracers-coronavirus-questions-answered-faq/; and Bryan Pietsch, "Coronavirus Tracers Beg Residents: Please Answer Your Phones," *New York Times*, September 29, 2020.

34. "Those Americans who": Dalton, "Contact Tracing, the West's Big Hope for Suppressing Covid-19," and Teo Armas, "Coronavirus Detectives Couldn't Get Partygoers to Answer the Phone. So They Issued Subpoenas," *Washington Post*, July 3, 2020. "Nor is this": Benjamin Mueller, "Contact Tracing, Key to Reining in the Virus, Falls Flat in the West," *New York Times*, October 3, 2020. "A third of": Olga Khazan, "The Most American COVID-19 Failure Yet," *Atlantic Monthly*, August 31, 2020, accessed October 2, 2020, https://www.theatlantic.com/politics/archive/2020/08/contact-tracing-hr-6666-working-us/615637/. "In one case": Armas, "Coronavirus Detectives."

35. "Researchers in the," "The respondents said," and "Men, young people": Louise Smith et al., "Adherence to the Test, Trace and Isolate System: Results from a Time Series of 21 Nationally Representative Surveys in the U.K. (the COVID-19 Rapid Survey of Adherence to Interventions and Responses [CORSAIR] Study)," September 18, 2020, https://www.medrxiv.org/content/10.1101/2020.09.15.20191957v1.full.pdf.

36. "Those who are": Thirty percent of people in the U.S. with household incomes below $30,000 a year don't own a smartphone; 14 percent of those with annual household incomes of less than $100,000 also don't own smartphones (Monica Anderson and Madhumitha Kumar, "Digital Divide Persists Even as Lower-Income Americans Make Gains in Tech Adoption," Pew Research Center, May 7, 2019, accessed September 13, 2020, https://www.pewresearch.org/fact-tank/2019/05/07/digital-divide-persists-even-as-lower-income-americans-make-gains-in-tech-adoption/). And, as in

Singapore, the elderly have been slower to adopt technology. In 2017 only 42 percent of Americans over sixty-five had smartphones (Monica Anderson and Andrew Perrin, "Tech Adoption Climbs among Older Adults," Pew Research Center, May 17, 2017, https://www.pewresearch.org/internet /2017/05/17/tech-adoption-climbs-among-older-adults/).

37. "In 2011, the": Government of the United Kingdom, "Isle of Wight 2011 Census Atlas," 15, accessed October 25, 2020, https://www.iow.gov .uk/azservices/documents/2552-Census-Atlas-2011-Section-2-Population -religion-and-ethnicity.pdf. "In Newham, by": National Health Service, Covid-19 app support, "Why Has the NHS Chosen Newham to Trial Their Contact Tracing App?," accessed October 7, 2020, https://faq.covid19.nhs .uk/article/KA-01215/en-us?parentid=CAT-01041&rootid=CAT-01021. "Residents of the": Sarah Boseley, "Take-Up of NHS Contact-Tracing App Could Be Only 10%," *Guardian*, September 24, 2020.

38. "They couldn't learn": Marcel Salathé, Christian L. Althaus, Nanina Anderegg, et al., "Early Evidence of Effectiveness of Digital Contact" (October 4, 2020), 7–8, https://www.medrxiv.org/content/10.1101/2020 .09.07.20189274v3.full.pdf, and Serge Vaudenay and Martin Vuagnoux, "The Dark Side of SwissCovid," https://lasec.epfl.ch/people/vaudenay/swiss covid.html#effectiveness. "They could learn": Ireland's Covid Tracker does collect such metrics if the user opts in; "Data Protection Information Notice COVID Tracker App," accessed October 9, 2020, https://covidtracker.gov .ie/privacy-and-data/data-protection.

39. "Earlier coronaviruses, like": Zhuang Shen, Fang Ning, Weigong Zhou, et al., "Superspreading SARS Events, Beijing, 2003," *Emerging Infectious Diseases* 10, no. 2 (February 2004): 256–260, and Hiroshi Nihkiura et al., "Identifying Determinants of Heterogeneous Transmission Dynamics of the Middle East Respiratory Syndrome (MERS) Outbreak in the Republic of Korea, 2015: A Retrospective Epidemiological Analysis," *BMJ Open* 6, no. 2 (2016). "The pattern for": Yunjun Zhang et al., "Evaluating Transmission Heterogeneity and Super-Spreading Event of COVID-19 in a Metropolis of China," *International Journal of Environmental Research and Public Health* 17, no. 10 (May 24, 2020); Max S. Y. Lau et al., "Characterizing Superspreading Events and Age-Specific Infectiousness of SARS-CoV-2 Transmission in Georgia, USA," *PNAS* 117, no. 26 (September 8, 2020); Agus Hasan et al., "Superspreading in Early Transmissions of COVID-19 in Indonesia," July 24, 2020, accessed October 9, 2020, https://www.medrxiv.org/content

/medrxiv/early/2020/07/24/2020.06.28.20142133.full; and Akira Endo, Sam Abbott, Adam J. Kucharski, and Sebastian Funk, "Estimating the Overdispersion in COVID-19 Transmission Using Outbreak Sizes outside China," accessed October 9, 2020, https://wellcomeopenresearch.org/articles/5-67/v3.

40. "Many infected people": Endo et al., "Estimating the Overdispersion." "Superspreading is most": Benjamin M. Althouse, Edward A. Wenger, Joel C. Miller, et al., "Stochasticity and Heterogeneity in the Transmission Dynamics of SARS-CoV-2," preprint, May 27, 2020, https://arxiv.org/pdf /2005.13689.pdf.

41. "Shefali Oza, Data": Shefali Oza (Data and Testing Manager, Partners in Health), interview with the author, June 12, 2020.

42. "The most likely": Philip Bump, "What We Know about the Timeline of the White House Coronavirus Cluster—And What We Don't," *Washington Post*, October 10, 2020.

43. "Though the two": Apple, "Exposure Notifications Frequently Asked Questions Preliminary Subject to Modification and Extension," v. 1.2, September 2020, accessed September 19, 2020, https://covid19-static.cdn -apple.com/applications/covid19/current/static/contact-tracing/pdf/Expo sureNotification-FAQv1.2.pdf.

44. "Common Circle, one": Justin Chan et al., "PACT: Privacy Sensitive Protocols and Mechanisms for Mobile Contact Tracing," May 7, 2020, 11, https://commoncircle.us/Whitepaper.html.

45. "The UK's NHS": Government of the United Kingdom, "Create a Coronavirus NHS QR Code for Your Venue," accessed October 14, 2020, https:// www.gov.uk/create-coronavirus-qr-poster. "If there's a": National Health Service, Government of the United Kingdom, "NHS COVID-19 App: An Introduction to QR Posters for Businesses," accessed October 14, 2020, https://www.youtube.com/watch?v=o09mQuvRMAQ.

Chapter 6

1. "But in the": Liza Lin, "China Marshals Its Surveillance Powers against Coronavirus; Officials Use Big Data to Track the Movements of Infected Individuals," *Wall Street Journal*, February 4, 2020; Kate Ng, "'Sharp-Tongued Drones' Chastise Chinese Residents for Not Wearing Face Masks amid Coronavirus Outbreak," *Independent*, January 31, 2020; and Paul

Mozur, "China, Desperate to Stop Coronavirus, Turns Neighbor against Neighbor," *New York Times*, February 3, 2020.

2. "In April 2020": Michael Veale, "Contact Tracing Protocols," in Linnet Taylor et al., eds., *Data Justice and COVID-19: Global Perspectives* (London: Meatspace Press, 2020), and European Parliament, "P9_TA(2020)0054 EU Coordinated Action to Combat the COVID-19 Pandemic and Its Consequences. European Parliament Resolution of 17 April 2020 on EU Coordinated Action to Combat the COVID-19 Pandemic and Its Consequences (2020/2616(RSP))," https://www.europarl.europa.eu/doceo/document/TA -9-2020-0054_EN.pdf.

3. "The apps infrastructure": Google, "Exposure Notification Frequently Asked Questions Preliminary—Subject to Modification and Extension," v. 1.2, July 2020, 5, https://blog.google/documents/73/Exposure_Notification _-_FAQ_v1.1.pdf.

4. "Google and Apple": Leo Kelion, "Coronavirus: First Google/Apple-Based Contact-Tracing App Launched," *BBC News*, May 28, 2020, https:// www.bbc.com/news/technology-52807635.

5. "This tool let": The menu included distance and length of exposure, user interface text, logos, URLs of follow-up sites, and other items. See Google, accessed October 13, 2020, https://github.com/google/exposure -notifications-android/blob/master/doc/enexpress-config.md, and Apple, "Configuring Exposure Notifications," accessed October 7, 2020, https:// developer.apple.com/documentation/exposurenotification/configuring _exposure_notifications#overview. "This tool let" and "'Public health wants'": Bill Darrow (Professor, Department of Health Promotion and Disease Prevention, Florida International University), interview with the author, September 18, 2020.

6. "First and foremost": Koustubh "K.J." Bagchi et al., *Digital Tools for COVID-19 Contact Tracing: Identifying and Mitigating the Equity, Privacy, and Civil Liberties Concerns*, Edmond Safra Center for Ethics, Open Technology Institute, and New America (July 2, 2020): 5–6; Ethics Advisory Board, NHSX, Letter to Secretary of State (April 24, 2020): 3, accessed October 18, 2020, https://nhsbsa-socialtracking.powerappsportals.com /EAB%20Letter%20to%20NHSx.pdf; Neema Singh Guiliani, ACLU, *Government Safeguards for Tech-Assisted Contact Tracing* (May 18, 2020), 2; and reports from multiple other organizations.

7. "Second, use of": Bagchi et al., *Digital Tools for COVID-19*, 13, 37, and 42; Ethics Advisory Board, Letter to Secretary of State, 3; Guiliani, *Government Safeguards*, 2–4; and reports from multiple other organizations. "The same goes": Government of Australia, Privacy Amendment (Public Health Contact Information) Act 2020, No. 44 (2020).

8. "Third, use of": Bagchi et al., *Digital Tools for COVID-19 Contact Tracing*, 36; Guiliani, *Government Safeguards*, 2. "Switzerland's Epidemic Act": Government of Switzerland, Bundesgesetz über die Bekämpfung übertragbarer Krankheiten des Menschen (Federal Law on Combating Communicable Diseases in Humans), Article 60a, abs 2. "Australia's 2020 Act": Government of Australia, Privacy Amendment.

9. "Fifth, policymakers should": Guiliani, *Government Safeguards*, 2; Ethics Advisory Board, Letter to Secretary of State, 3; and reports from multiple other organizations. "That means that": Chaos Computer Club, "10 Requirements for the Evaluation of 'Contact Tracing' Apps," April 6, 2020, https://www.ccc.de/en/updates/2020/contact-tracing-requirements.

10. "So far, various": Johanna Stern, "Curbing Coronavirus with a Contact-Tracing App? It's Not So Simple," *Wall Street Journal*, May 9, 2020, and "Jumbo Privacy Review: North Dakota's Contact Tracing App," Jumbo blog, https://blog.jumboprivacy.com/jumbo-privacy-review-north-dakota -s-contact-tracing-app.html, May 21, 2020. "At one point": Aroon Deep, "Aarogya Setu Vulnerability Gave Up Users' Precise Location Data to Google," *Medianama*, April 27, 2020. "An error in": Alex Hern, "Fault in NHS Covid app meant thousands at risk did not quarantine," *Guardian*, November 2, 2020. "Google and Apple": This recommendation appears in Bagchi et al., *Digital Tools for COVID-19 Contact Tracing*, 42.

11. "Google and Apple": In June 2020, two US senators, Maria Cantwell and Bill Cassidy, introduced a bill addressing the privacy of app information (Exposure Notification Privacy Act, 116th Congress, 2nd Session, https:// www.cantwell.senate.gov/imo/media/doc/Exposure%20Notification%20 Privacy%20Bill%20Text.pdf).

12. "Only governments are": This is a point made by various organizations and scholars; see, e.g., Bagchi et al., *Digital Tools for COVID-19 Contact Tracing*, 39.

13. "All but two": K. H. Kim et al., "Middle East Respiratory Syndrome Coronavirus (MERS-CoV) Outbreak in South Korea, 2015: Epidemiology,

Characteristics, and Public Health Implications," *Journal of Hospital Infection* 95, no. 2 (2017), and David S. Hui, Stanley Perlman, and Alimuddin Zumla, "Spread of MERS to South Korea and China," *The Lancet Respiratory Medicine* 3, no. 7 (July 1, 2015): 509–510. "Nor did the": Alastair Gale and Kwanwoo Jun, "Korea's MERS Outbreak Highlights SARS Lessons; Experts Cite the Need for a Quick Quarantine and Public Disclosure," *Wall Street Journal*, June 10, 2015.

14. "When COVID-19 hit": Ministry of Science and ICT, Republic of Korea, *How We Fought COVID-19: A Perspective from Science and ICT* (July 2020): 10–11.

15. "In 2015, however": Ministry of Science and ICT, *How We Fought COVID-19*, 26. Note that the Korea Centers for Disease Control and Prevention was restructured in September 2020 and the organization's name was changed to the Korea Disease Control and Prevention Agency.

16. "Some were stigmatized": Choe Sung-Han, "In South Korea, Covid-19 Comes with Another Risk: Online Bullies," *New York Times*, October 2, 2020, and Nemo Kim, "'More Scary than Coronavirus': South Korea's Health Alerts Expose Private Lives," *Guardian*, March 5, 2020.

17. "After several such": Sung-Han, "In South Korea."

18. "In 2012, after": The search was limited to email headers, to determine if someone had forwarded mail. To many this was a distinction without a difference. Richard Perez-Peña, "Harvard Search of E-Mail Stuns Its Faculty Members," *New York Times*, March 10, 2013. "That the search": In fact, such information can be remarkably revelatory. See, e.g., Jonathan Mayer, Patrick Mutchler, and John C. Mitchell, "Evaluating the Privacy Properties of Telephone Metadata," *PNAS* 113, no. 20 (May 17, 2016): 5536–5541; Steven M. Bellovin et al., "It's Too Complicated: How the Internet Upends *Katz, Smith*, and Electronic Surveillance Law," *Harvard Journal of Law and Technology* 30, no. 1 (2017); and Susan Landau, "Categorizing Uses of Communications Metadata: Systematizing Knowledge and Presenting a Path for Privacy," New Security Paradigms Workshop, 2020.

19. "Aside from routine": Harvard University, "Policy on Access to Electronic Information, as Voted by the President and Fellows of Harvard College on March 31, 2014; Amended May 8, 2015," accessed October 15, 2020, https://hwpi.harvard.edu/files/provost/files/policy_on_access_to_elec tronic_information.pdf.

20. "The university had": Harvard University, "Coronavirus Main: Testing and Tracing," accessed October 17, 2020, https://www.harvard.edu/corona virus/testing-tracing#unobserved. "With this system" and "Once you've decided": "Tracking Covid at U.S. Colleges and Universities," *New York Times*, October 8, 2020, accessed October 15, 2020, https://www.nytimes .com/interactive/2020/us/covid-college-cases-tracker.html.

21. "But if we've": Nate Anderson, "How 'Cell Tower Dumps' Caught the High Country Bandits—And Why It Matters," Ars Technica, August 29, 2013, and Susan Landau, *Listening In: Cybersecurity in an Insecure Age* (New Haven, CT: Yale University Press), 131–132. In 2020, two federal magistrates pushed back against such practices on the grounds of the searches being too broad and lacking sufficient particularization; see United States District Court for the Northern District of Illinois Eastern Division, "In the Matter of the Search of: Information Stored at Premises Controlled by Google, as Further Described in Attachment A, Case No. 20 M 297 Magistrate Judge M. David Weisman, July 8, 2020" and the United States District Court for the Northern District of Illinois Eastern Division, "In the Matter of the Search of: Information Stored at Premises Controlled by Google, No 20 M 392, Honorable Gabriel A. Fuentes, U.S. Magistrate Judge," August 24, 2020.

22. "A 1993 National": National Research Council, *The Social Impact of AIDS in the United States* (Washington, DC: National Academies Press, 1993), 1. "COVID-19 has produced": Public Health England, *Disparities in the Risk and Outcomes of COVID-19*, August 2020, 6; Anne-Diandra Louarn, "Death Tolls Show France's Immigrants Hardest Hit by COVID-19, Study Finds," INFOMIGRANTS, July 17, 2020, accessed October 17, 2020, https://www.infomigrants.net/en/post/26034/death-tolls-show-france-s -immigrants-hardest-hit-by-covid-19-study-finds; and Shabani Mahtani, "Singapore Lost Control of Its Coronavirus Outbreak, and Migrant Workers Are the Victims," *Washington Post*, April 21, 2020.

23. "The apps are": Brittlestar, "Should You Really Get the Covid Alert App?," 1:14–1:35, accessed October 17, 2020, https://twitter.com/brittlestar /status/1317166286221303809. "But you can't": Chas Kissick, "Privacy Issues at the Heart of North Carolina's Coronavirus, Response," *Lawfare*, October 15, 2020.

SELECTED BIBLIOGRAPHY

This is a brief list of references; many more, especially research papers, can be found in the endnotes.

Books

Brandt, Allan M. *No Magic Bullet: A Social History of Venereal Disease in the United States since 1880, with a New Chapter on AIDS.* Oxford: Oxford University Press, 1987.

Brilliant, Lawrence B. *The Management of Smallpox Eradication in India: A Case Study and Analysis.* Ann Arbor: University of Michigan Press, June 1, 1985.

Conlon, Richard T. *From the Merry Widow Bar To . . . : Tales of a Venereal Disease Investigator during the 1960s and 1970s.* Self-published, 2019.

de Kruif, Paul. *Microbe Hunters, with a New Introduction by F. Gonzalez-Crussi.* New York: Harcourt, Brace, 1996.

Foege, William H. *House on Fire: The Fight to Eradicate Smallpox.* Berkeley: University of California Press, 2011.

Johns Hopkins Project on Ethics and Governance of Digital Contact Tracing Technologies. *Digital Contact Tracing for Pandemic Research: Ethics and Governance Guidance.* Baltimore: Johns Hopkins University Press, 2020.

Jones, James H. *Bad Blood: The Tuskegee Syphilis Experiment.* New and expanded ed. New York: Free Press, 1993.

Leavitt, Judith Walzer. *Typhoid Mary: Captive to the Public Health.* Boston: Beacon Press, 1996.

Meyerson, Beth E., Fred A. Martich, and Gerald P. Naehr. *Ready to Go: The History and Contributions of U.S. Public Health Advisors*. Research Triangle Park, NC: American Social Health Association, 2008.

Parran, Thomas. *Shadow on the Land: Syphilis*. New York: Reynal and Hitchcock, 1937.

Potterat, John J. *Seeking the Positives: A Life Spent on the Cutting Edge of Public Health*. Self-published, 2015.

Shilts, Randy. *And the Band Played On: Politics, People, and the AIDS Epidemic*. New York: St. Martin's Griffin, 1988.

Taylor, Linnet, Gargi Sharma, Aaron Martin, and Shazade Jameson, eds. *Data Justice and COVID-19: Global Perspectives*. London: Meatspace Press, 2020.

Tomes, Nancy. *The Gospel of Germs: Men, Women, and the Microbe in American Life*. Cambridge, MA: Harvard University Press, 1998.

Wachtler, Robert. *The Digital Doctor: Hope, Hype, and Harm at the Dawn of Medicine's Computer Age*. New York: McGraw Hill, 2017.

Reports

Ad Hoc Pandemic-Response Subgroup of Former Members of President Obama's Council of Advisors on Science and Technology. *The Role of Contact Tracing in the Control of Microbial Epidemics, Including COVID-19*, June 18, 2020, http://opcast.org/OPCAST_On_Contact_Tracing_06-18-20.pdf.

Bagchi, Koustubh "K.J.," Christine Bannan, Sharon Bradford Franklin, Heather Hurlburt, Lauren Sarkesian, Ross Schulman, and Joshua Stager. *Digital Tools for COVID-19 Contact Tracing: Identifying and Mitigating the Equity, Privacy, and Civil Liberties Concerns*, Edmond Safra Center for Ethics, Open Technology Institute, and New America, July 2, 2020.

Hinch, Robert, Will Probert, Anel Nurtay, Michelle Kendall, Chris Wymant, Matthew Hall, Katrina Lythgoe, Ana Bulas Cruz, Lele Zhao, Andrea Stewart, et al. *Effective Configurations of Digital Contact-Tracing Apps: A Report to NHSX*, April 16, 2020, accessed October 18, 2020, https://cdn.theconversation.com/static_files/files/1009/Report_-_Effective_App_Configurations.pdf?1587531217.

Ministry of Science and ICT, Republic of Korea. *How We Fought COVID-19: A Perspective from Science and ICT*, July 2020.

Websites and Videos

Darrow, William. Interview on *The Early Years of AIDS: CDC's Response to a Historic Epidemic*, https://www.globalheathchronicles.org/items/show /6870, November 21, 2016.

Gurley, Emily. "COVID-19 Contact Tracing," Johns Hopkins University Coursera Course, accessed July 14, 2020, https://www.coursera.org/learn /covid-19-contact-tracing?edocomorp=covid-19-contact-tracing.

Papers and Articles

Budd, J., B. S. Miller, E. M. Manning, et al. "Digital Technologies in the Public-Health Response to COVID-19." *Nature Medicine* 26 (2020): 1183–1192. https://doi.org/10.1038/s41591-020-1011-4.

Coltart, C. E., B. Lindsey, I. Ghinai, A. M. Johnson, and D. L. Heymann. "The Ebola Outbreak, 2013–2016: Old Lessons for New Epidemics." *Philosophical Transactions of the Royal Society of London. Series B, Biological Sciences* 372, no. 1721 (2017): 20160297. https://doi.org/10.1098/rstb.2016.0297.

Duhigg, Charles. "Seattle's Leaders Let Scientists Take the Lead. New York Did Not." *New Yorker*, May 4, 2020.

Stern, Joanna, and Kenny Wassus. "How Coronavirus-Tracking Apps Work." *Wall Street Journal*, September 17, 2020, accessed September 17, 2020, https://www.wsj.com/articles/contact-tracing-the-wests-big-hope-for -suppressing-covid-19-is-in-disarray-11600337670.

Tufecki, Zeynep. "This Overlooked Variable Is the Key to the Pandemic." *Atlantic*, September 30, 2020.

INDEX

and location tracking, 57–58
policies, 70
and proximity data, 54–55,
    58–59, 61, 68–74
and security, 71–74
and sexual partners, 13, 14
and well-known people, 68–69
Privacy-protective technology,
    59–62
Protozoans, 1, 2
Proximity data, 54–55, 58–74
Public Health Advisers (PHAs),
    22–25, 30
Public health
    distrust of, 91
    distrust of by Black Americans,
        20, 22

QR code, 97
Quarantine, 13, 14, 18, 42, 54, 69,
    76, 102. *See also* Isolation
    China, 13, 99
    Ebola, 32, 34
    India, 50
    Mary Mallon, 13
    South Korea, 35, 36, 42
    Switzerland, 93
    Wuhan, 13

R_0 (R naught), 7–8
    and contact tracing, 75, 87
Racism
    and contact tracing, 82–87
    Tuskegee study, 20–22, 24
Rats, and bubonic plague, 6
Redi, Francisco, 2–3
Reynolds, Stewart, 109

Rothenberg, Richard, 62
RSA meeting, 117n2

SafeEntry (Singapore), 48
Salvarsan, 20
Sana, Ibn, 2
San Francisco, Department of
    Public Health, 25
Sanitation, and pandemics, 8–9
SARS, 94
SARS-CoV-2, 9, 36. *See also*
    Coronavirus
Security, and privacy, 71–74
Sencer, David, 24
Seoul, South Korea, 38
Sexually transmitted diseases
    (STDs), 13, 20
    chancroid, 20
    HIV/AIDS, 13, 109 (*see also*
        HIV/AIDS)
    gonorrhea, 13, 20
    syphilis, 12, 19–20, 57 (*see also*
        Syphilis)
Shin Bet (Israel), 40–41
Shincheonji Church of Jesus (South
    Korea), 37
Sickels, Ryane, 29
Singapore
    contact tracing in 44–48, 54, 90,
        99
    Ministry of Health (MOH),
        44–45, 54, 62
    and privacy, 54–55
    SafeEntry, 48
    TraceTogether app (Singapore),
        44–48, 51, 53–54, 71, 96, 99,
        103

Indian Health Service, 88–89
National Academies of Science, 109
Office of Personnel Management, 72
public health, as responsibility of states and local governments in, 67
Public Health Service (USPHS), 21, 22, 25
University of Dublin, 78
University of Miami, Miller School of Medicine, 86–87
University of Oxford, 47

Vaccination
  cowpox, 10
  smallpox, 10–11, 16
van Leeuwenhoek, Antonie, 3
Virginia (state), 67, 80, 101
Viruses, 1, 2. *See also* Coronavirus; Ebola; HIV/AIDS; Middle East respiratory syndrome (MERS); SARS; SARS-CoV-2; Smallpox; West Nile virus
  mutations in, 5–6

Wall Street Journal, 90
Washington (state), contract tracing apps in, 42, 67–68
Washington Post, 95
West Nile virus, 9
White House, COVID-19 outbreak in, 94–95
White Mountain Apache Tribe, 87–89, 92
Whiteriver Indian Hospital, 88

Wi Fi networks, used for contact tracing and exposure notification, 42–43, 104, 107
World Health Organization (WHO), 11, 38
  and Ebola, 33
Wuhan, quarantine, 13

Yasnine, Willis Archie, 33–34
Yersinia pestis, 6

Zoonotic diseases, 5–6, 9
  MERS, 34